MOST OF WHAT YOU KNOW ABOUT **ADDICTION IS WRONG**

Anirudh Kala

Foreword by **Dr Atul Ambekar, Professor,**
National Drug Dependence Treatment Centre
& Department of Psychiatry, AIIMS, New Delhi

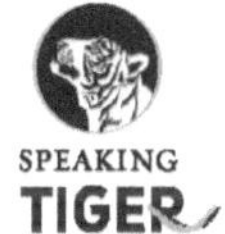

SPEAKING TIGER BOOKS LLP
125A, Ground Floor, Shahpur Jat, near Asiad Village,
New Delhi 110049

First published by Speaking Tiger Books 2023

ISBN: 978-93-5447-465-1
eISBN: 978-93-5447-446-0

10 9 8 7 6 5 4 3 2 1

Anirudh Kala is a psychiatrist by profession. He is Clinical Director of Mind Plus, an intermediate stay facility for treatment of substance use disorders at Ludhiana, Punjab. Kala was a member of the expert group tasked by the Government of India with writing mental health policy for the country, which was released in 2014. He has been instrumental in forging cross-border links between mental health professionals of Indian and Pakistani Punjab provinces and is the founder of the Indo-Pak Punjab Psychiatric Society.

Kala also writes fiction. He is the author of the short story collection, *Unsafe Asylum: Stories of Partition and Madness* (Speaking Tiger Books, 2018) and the novel, *Two and a Half Rivers* (Niyogi Books, 2021).

He is fond of Urdu poetry, travel and photography.

CONTENTS

Foreword

As an addiction psychiatrist, I have been looking for a comprehensive, authoritative and yet easy-to-read book for common readers on addictions and India. I found it rather strange that in this large and diverse country of ours—with a good number (not enough though) of professionals with the required level of knowledge of the subject—there is no single source of information on the history of our tryst with addictive drugs as well as our ongoing love-hate relationship with them. The popular rhetoric of a 'drug-free world' notwithstanding, this book elegantly introduces us to the way Indians have been engaging with addictive substances. As today's youngsters prefer to call some of their relationships—'it's complicated'.

Professor Anirudh Kala is very well-known among the psychiatry fraternity in India. His books of fiction, taking a cue from the recent history of Punjab with the backdrop of the Partition (*Unsafe Asylum: Stories of Partition and Madness*) and militancy (*Two and a Half Rivers*) have been creating ripples. In *Most of What You Know About Addiction Is Wrong*, he turns his attention to the much talked about but largely misunderstood topic of addictions. While for understandable reasons the addiction situation in Punjab figures prominently here, it will be unfair to say that this is a book about addictions in Punjab. This is a book about addictions. Period.

The book begins where it all started—with the early humans, their initial forays into 'civilization' and the establishment of their relationship with mind-altering substances. Subsequently, Professor Kala shares a rich and entertaining historical account of the use of various substances in Indian society through different periods in history (with more focus on the recent past, of course). Apart from the history of addictions, Professor Kala also describes the science of addictions. The nature-versus-nurture debate about the origins of addictions has been dexterously handled in the book.

A highlight of *Most of What You Know About Addiction Is Wrong* is the way data has been treated. Statistics about the number of people using drugs and those affected by addictions have not just been quoted but explained in an easy-to-understand manner. The book draws the reader's attention towards the criticality of credible data on substance use and skilfully demonstrates how to derive meaning from that data.

Interspersed throughout *Most of What You Know About Addiction Is Wrong* are key messages about how a mature society should handle addictive drugs. The book exhorts policymakers to shun the *war* on drugs and instead seriously consider making *peace* with drugs. As Kofi Annan, former Secretary General of the United Nations put it, 'Drugs have destroyed many lives, but wrong government policies have destroyed many more.' Wish our policymakers would take note. Meanwhile, the pursuit to enhance our understanding of addictions and effective ways to deal with them must continue.

—Dr Atul Ambekar

Professor, National Drug Dependence
Treatment Centre and Department of Psychiatry,
All India Institute of Medical Sciences, New Delhi and
Secretary General, Addiction Psychiatry Society of India

CHAPTER 1

Human Beings and Drugs Are Evolutionary Companions

The histories of humankind and opium are intimately intertwined. We have been using narcotic drugs for about 10,000 years both as medicines and as intoxicants. About 10,000 years ago, our hunter-gatherer ancestors started settling down for the first time in an area which we now know as West Asia, to live in groups, sow crops and tend to cattle. This is also the place where much later, the first cities were built and organized trade, study of science, mathematics, philosophy and the arts originated. Three major religions of the world would also start from here. The first opium plant, carbon dated and estimated to be 8,000 years old was also found here (in the Jordan Valley).

The first evidence of opium addiction in humans was discovered in Spain when a 7500-year-old skeleton was found with the residue of a poppy pod stuck in its teeth and the analysis of the bones indicated years of opium consumption. In 1989 archaeologists found evidence of a large settlement dating back 7,000 years near Rome. From the remains and the articles found they concluded that this was a colony of people from another civilization—in all probability from across the Mediterranean. Findings included seeds of the opium plant,

Papaver somniferum. This could have been the way opium reached Europe from the Middle East.

Around the same time, brewing of beer had begun in what is now modern-day Iraq and adjoining areas. So, the early Bronze Age humans already had two of the major intoxicants that we have today i.e., alcohol and opium, and that too in a geographical area where alcohol is at present taboo as it is strictly banned for religious reasons. Opium and opioid drugs continue to be the most effective pain relievers known to modern man. It is worth noting that 7,000 years back, severe pain whether from toothache, childbirth or battle injuries, could be alleviated almost as effectively as it can be today.

Caves in Spain have revealed 4,000-year-old burial chambers with bodies wearing elaborate gold jewellery buried along with poppy capsules encased in specially woven bags, which also contain locks of hair indicating that some type of ceremony was involved. This shows that opium poppy was being venerated ritually in some ancient societies of Europe (Inglis, 2018).

In a museum on the Greek island of Crete stands a 3,500-year-old 'goddess of poppy' statue wearing three hairpins of poppy capsules on her head. Arms raised, eyes closed and sporting a mystic expression, she looks to be under the effect of a drug. A clay pipe big enough to have sufficed for communal use was also found there and according to Inglis, this is probably the first drug apparatus in history and the first indication that opium was already being used not just for medicinal but also for recreational and relaxation purposes.

A 3,500-year-old papyrus found by a tomb raider on a mummy in Egypt contains detailed instructions on how to dose infants with opium. For thousands of years, parents all over the world routinely used opium to soothe crying infants. This practice has abated only in the last couple of hundred years.

Marcus Aurelius was the emperor of Rome in the 2nd century AD. Galen, his personal physician, used to accompany the emperor on his battle campaigns. He gave him a mixture of various ingredients one of which was opium, to tide over the rigours of battle. When the emperor appeared drowsy, he would skip the opium component but then the emperor did not sleep. Galen noted that, 'he was obliged to have recourse to poppy juice [for the emperor] since this was now "habitual" with him' (Inglis, 2018). Emperor Marcus Aurelius is considered to be possibly the first documented person in history addicted to opium although addiction as a concept was not understood then.

There were already large-scale travel and trade interactions between Persia and China and as part of those exchanges, opium seeds and product were brought to China from the Middle East in the late 6th or early 7th century. As far as tobacco is concerned it was the Spanish who took it to China. The Chinese loved tobacco despite the harsh edicts mandating ear mutilation for smoking. Women smoked tobacco as well as opium inside their houses and an official Chinese document in 1701 reported, 'From officials to servants and women everyone smokes today' (Inglis, 2018).

Between the 3rd and 6th century BC, poppy appeared on coins in Turkey and Rome. This was also the period of the massive victorious sweep by Alexander the Great. He is occasionally credited with bringing opium and its seeds to India. References to opium are not available in the Vedas, Puranas and not even in early Ayurvedic classics such as *Charka Samhita* (3rd to 2nd century BC), *Sushruta Samhita* (5th to 4th century BC) or any other medical treatise of the time (Dwarka Nath, 1965).

Only after the 14th century, opium was openly mentioned

as a component of several medications. It is highly probable therefore that opium came to India three to four hundred years before the Mohammedan conquests in the 9th-10th century AD and not with Alexander's army. Arab traders were coming to India even before the armies did and opium could very well have been brought by them in the 7th century. What is well known is that it was extensively used by Hindu physicians in the 15th century.

On the other hand, cannabis is mentioned much earlier than opium in almost all the medical texts of antiquity implying that while opium came from outside, cannabis is either native to India or was brought to India from central Asia by the Aryans around 2000 BC. According to a legend, Lord Shiva himself is said to have brought cannabis down from Mount Kailash for the pleasure of mankind.

Both *Atharvaveda* and *Sushruta Samhita* mention bhang as one of the five sacred plants that relieve anxiety. Lord Shiva is said to be particularly fond of cannabis products like bhang and ganja and on Shivratri, for his birth celebrations, the devout in large swathes of North and East India ceremonially consume bhang and charas. This is over and above the regular use by a large number of people in the states of UP, Bihar, Rajasthan, Orissa, Assam and West Bengal. According to Dwarka Nath (1965), 'Bona fide religious mendicants make use of cannabis, especially ganja, which they smoke as an aid to their meditation, concentration and other religious practices. This practice can be traced to a period earlier than the 17th century AD.'

The Marathi poet, Madhva Munishwara in 1733 AD, describing the life of *yogis* and *jangamas* (nomadic mendicants), noted that they were addicted to cannabis–especially ganja and opium. The practice continues in many religious ashrams.

According to a *Times of India* report of September 7, 2020, some temples and *mutts* in Karnataka give marijuana as *prasad* (holy offering) to devotees as it 'helps in meditation'.

The hippy trail in the sixties came to India via Kabul and then spread out to Srinagar, Kathmandu, Delhi, Mumbai and Goa. The hippies who flocked to India were seeking not only cannabis but an alternate lifestyle of which cannabis was a part. They found this in the ashrams and villages along the Ganga. Many immersed themselves in the Hindu religion and within a few years, mysticism, meditation and Indian clothes came to be popular among the youth in the West.

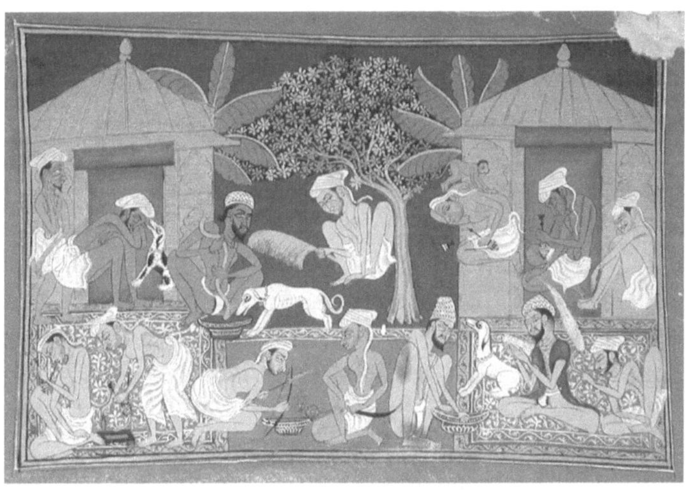

'Bhang Eaters in Front of Two Huts', The San Diego Museum of Art, Edwin Binney 3rd Collection. (*Wikimedia Commons*)

As far as the use of alcohol among the ancient Hindus is concerned, Dr Rajendralala Mitra, in a scholarly paper published in the Asiatic Society's Journal (Volume XLII, Part I, 1873, quoted in 'A History of the Excise System in the Punjab: 1846-

1884' by Raj Kishan Kapur, 1931) shows conclusively, by a profusion of instances taken from Sanskrit literature—ancient and medieval, that spirits and other intoxicating drinks have been extensively used in India at all times and by all classes. He states that their use was condemned by moralists and lawmakers, but rice-spirit was sold and drunk, and used in sacrifices in the earliest Vedic times. In the time of Kalidasa, drinking seems to have been very common not only among men but even among women of high rank.

~

Ottoman sultans took opium as a matter of course and people rationalized it generously on the grounds that being Muslims, they did not drink, implying some intoxicant was in order.

The second great empire of the time was in Persia. John Chardin, a jeweller from France wrote about the capital, '...magnificent palaces, smiling houses, spacious caravanserais, very fine canals and bazars.' He also wrote that despite the strict Shiite Muslim ideology perhaps nine out of ten Persian men took opium pills (Chardin, 1673-77).

However, according to Inglis, '...it was towards the East that lay the most ostentatious opium eaters of all, the Mughal Emperors.' By the time the Mughals were established, the ruling classes of all three major empires of the world had cultivated a strong opium habit. But unlike the Ottoman and the Safavid emperors of Persia and despite their religion, the Mughals liked to drink wine too. Actually, a great deal of it. Inglis notes, 'Women were also allowed to join the parties although it is not certain if they were permitted to drink or partake just opium... from the tales of their feasting, carousing, eating and hunting, the Mughals were consumers on a tremendous scale. Humayun admitted freely of being an opium eater as was his son Akbar after him.'

The fact that the use of opium was prevalent in the time of Akbar is shown by references made to it by Abul Fazl in his *Ain-i-Akbari.* He states that even the emperor occasionally (one dare not write more in the official biography of an emperor) indulged in taking opium and kuknar, a beverage prepared from the poppy capsule. He observes that most of the nobility of the court of Akbar and Jahangir used a beverage composed of a mixture of hemp, opium and wine called char-burgha. However, by some accounts, both Humayun and Akbar paled in comparison to Jahangir in the amounts consumed. Jahangir remained so inebriated by his drinking and opium habits that from 1611 onwards his wife Nur Jahan practically ruled in his stead after his first wife Man Bai killed herself with an opium overdose in 1605. Both of Jehangir's brothers died of alcoholism.

The accounts of European travellers indicate that in the 16th century, Indians took opium on a large scale. This was mostly in the form of a drink called kusumba, or else it was eaten, but usually not smoked. Mostly, crude opium purchased from excise shops was used. However, no excise records are available to show the extent to which the use existed prior to 1857 when the cultivation of opium was brought under the control of the British Indian Government.

~

In the 17th century, London physician Thomas Sydenham made for his patients a liquid concoction called laudanum, which contained opium dissolved in alcohol. It would be later called 'tincture opii' by pharmacists. It was a raging success and soon became available in apothecaries across the counter and was touted as 'a rapidly intoxicating, fever-reducing painkiller that also calmed the bowels and the senses'. Sydenham's laudanum recipe was disseminated rapidly through England, western Europe and soon in America (Inglis, 2018). The use of laudanum was endemic, and it was taken by all classes of people for cough, diarrhoea, aches and pains, and as a sedative and for relaxation.

Two things happened around this time which fast forwarded the use and the ease of getting high on opium several times over:

1. Morphine which is a natural component of opium and is responsible for most although not all of its effects on the brain, was isolated from opium for the first time. Morphine, weight for weight, is ten times stronger than opium.

2. The injection syringe was invented and while it revolutionized administration of a large number of medications to very sick, injured and unconscious patients, injections of morphine too became possible and took the whole matter of opiate addiction to another level. By 1880, doctors in England and Europe realized that no medical discovery had been at the same time so great a blessing and so big a curse to mankind as the injection of morphine.

In America, the two opium preparations which became household names were Godfrey's cordial and Mrs Winslow's soothing syrup. Both were advertized as products for teething children to 'relieve the little sufferer at once' who would sleep and then awake 'bright as a button'. The advertisements carried pictures of beautiful, relaxed mothers and happy, round-cheeked children. Godfrey's cordial was plain tincture opii. Mrs Winslow's soothing syrup contained over 60 mgm of morphine per fluid ounce (29.57 ml).

America in those years was a predominantly rural country and distances were vast. Then came the mail order, equivalent of today's Amazon, and it made things far too easy for consumers. They just had to send money to the address given at the bottom

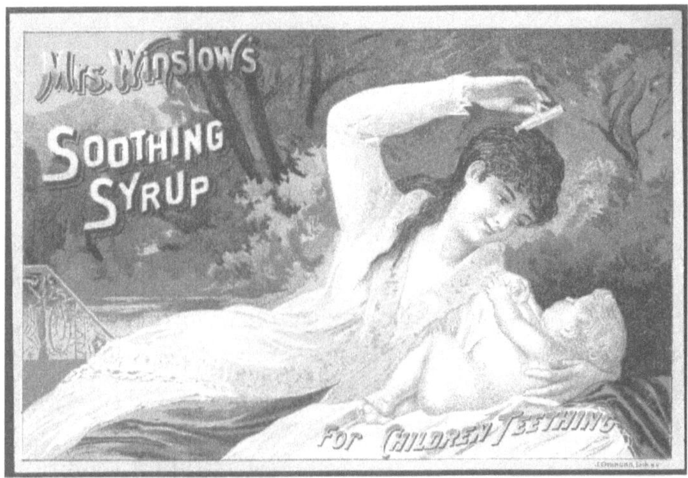

Advertisement for Mrs Winslow's Soothing Syrup. (*Wikimedia Commons*)

of the ad. No prescriptions were required. Also, men were moving from farmland in villages to factories in distant cities leaving their wives behind to look after their children. Tired and bored, with liquid opiates at hand, the mothers would take them too. Soon, the mail orders doubled and then quadrupled.

There is no doubt that just these two-opium based household remedies were the cause of not just relief from common ailments like pains, cough, diarrhoea and sleep disorders but were also of recreational use and resulted in a low to moderate level dependence on a fairly large scale in 19th- and early 20th-century America. Even then, today's addiction experts and progressive policy makers describe those times with a degree of romantic nostalgia, looking back it as a phase when intoxicants were mild, legal and easily available.

~

China had been sending its tea to Britain and Europe via the silk routes in central Asia, where it was in great demand not just as a casual drink but also as part of the typical British high tea ritual, which included elaborate tea sets, cakes, scones and biscuits. Soon tea became the staple drink of not just the rich and upper middleclass Britishers but also of the working people. Later, tea started being shipped from China to Britain on the ships of the East India Company (EIC). Very soon, the British were drinking more tea than the country could afford. The Chinese government did not fancy any British goods in exchange as payment for the Chinese tea consumed by the British. So, the tea had to be paid for in bullion, leading to a massive trade deficit which did not augur well for the British economy.

At the same time, the Chinese continued to consume vast amounts of opium most of which was supplied by the EIC despite it being illegal in China. The Company ferried it to China either from the Middle East or from India by sea which made it less competitive because the competition to supply opium to China was then from their co-Europeans, the Dutch. The Dutch ruled Malay Archipelago (now Indonesia) which was nearer to Chinese ports. In a historical twist of irony, two Christian superpowers of Europe were competing to sell opium to people of a heathen country in which trading and consumption of opium was strictly illegal and opium addiction rampant.

However, in 1757, the EIC tilted the scales of that competition hugely in Britain's favour by defeating Nawab Siraj-ud-Daulah of Bengal at the battle of Plassey, as the first step. The British did this by bribing Mir Jaffer, the Nawab's commander-in-chief with an offer of making him the Nawab after the battle. Bengal produced cheap and good quality opium which could now be packed in the factories of Patna and Benares and shipped from Calcutta to Canton in China much faster. Now, Britain could pay China for all the tea the British households drank with money obtained from selling Indian opium to Chinese traders.

As an aside, Robert Clive, who led the EIC to victory at Plassey, was himself a lifelong opium consumer. Later, back home in England, when faced with charges of massive corruption during his stay in India, he took an overdose of opium and cut his own throat in his home in Shropshire.

The massive illegal influx of opium into China led to the reversal of its trade surplus and created millions of opium addicts in the country which decreased the country's productivity. China issued an even starker prohibition order and confiscated millions of pounds of opium in weight, which had been ferried to China from India by British ships. The financial implications of this order sent shivers down the spines of British economists. The country responded by sending the Royal Navy to China in what was later known as The First Opium War (1839-42), which the British won hands down and compelled China to open its ports, so the British could resume smuggling their Indian opium to Chinese traders. As a bonus, the extortionate treaty they forced on China gave Hong Kong Island to the British Empire. It is sobering to note that Hong Kong and Shanghai Banking Corporation (HSBC), one of the largest banks operating in the word today, started by moving and managing opium money generated from the enforced sale of Indian opium by the British to a reluctant China. The Second Opium War (1856-60) was fought by the British and the French against China to extort even more commercial privileges and territorial concessions from China.

The unsavoury process by which Indian opium was dumped

onto China by the British using military force, had its moral rumblings in Britain. There was also the embarrassment the Christian missionaries in China doing their godly work had to face. When they advised their followers and potential converts to Christianity not to take opium, they were told to ask their country to stop supplying it first. Unsurprisingly, a moral uprising in Britain, demanding a stop to pushing Indian opium into China was led by Evangelicals and Quakers. This ultimately led to the formation of a Royal Commission on Opium in 1895, to study and report if the trade of Indian opium to China should be halted and also whether cultivation and consumption of opium in India itself should be banned for the good of the Indian population.

In addition to hundreds of administrators, social workers, lay persons and opium users, 111 medical experts were interviewed from all over the country. Two years later the nine-member Royal Commission consisting of seven English and two Indian members, answered both these questions in an unequivocal manner in a thousand-page report:

1. Concerns and protests of China were based on commercial considerations and not medical evidence.

2. Opium use in Asians (including China and India) was analogous to alcohol use in Europe and opium was not harmful to Asians.

The Commission also concluded that the habitual use of opium does not affect longevity. In his evidence before the Commission, MacLauchlan Slater, Manager, Actuary and Founder of the Oriental Government Security Life Assurance Company engaged in the business of insuring native lives told the Commission that based on their twenty years of research and experience they had not considered it necessary to place an extra premium on the lives of opium eaters!

After listening to conflicting views of experts on the effect of opium on a person's ability to reproduce, a member wryly noted, 'There is certainly no lack of fecundity in India.' The Commission dwelt at length on the use of opium in infants, which they noted was of ancient origin. Sometimes, suckling mothers smeared their nipples with small amounts of opium. 'Children's pills' or 'bala-golis' of two different strengths were available freely in markets. The practice was more prevalent with working women who put the infant in a basket next to their sites of work, but also very common in 'zenanas of the rich' because opium not only took care of persistent crying, it also prevented diarrhoea, soothed teething children and according to a staunchly held belief, helped in the digestion of milk.

Accidental overdosages did happen but 'very rarely and most infants recovered'. The Commission concluded, 'It is difficult to believe that a practice so widely diffused through all grades of society and carried on under the direct supervision of the vigilant maternal instinct should have maintained itself so long in credit, if it were on the whole and to any appreciable extent injurious.' A section of Shia Muslims called Bohras did not give opium to their children. A British doctor testifying before the commission at Indore said of their children, 'They happen to be the most unhealthy children in this part of the country... Whether it is from not taking opium, I do not know but as a matter of fact, the children of Bohras are very unhealthy!'

The Commission also noted in its report the accounts of ceremonial use of opium in the protected states of Rajputana, Central India and Gujarat during religious festivals, on state occasions, at marriage celebrations, at births and funerals, as a token of welcome to friends and as a seal of reconciliation between adversaries. A preparation called amalpani was used on such occasions.

Lastly, the Royal Opium Commission examined witnesses about the practice of smoking opium in the Indian population and concluded that smoking was far less common than oral intake and unlike in China, it was a subordinate habit. In India, smoking opium was more of a social activity among the not so well to do. Two preparations called madak and chandu were smoked; madak in the ordinary hubble-bubble pipe and chandu in specially made pipes, in which a bowl-shaped container made of terracotta containing chandu was fixed into a hole in a twenty-inch-long bamboo pipe, which was passed around. Chandu was roughly twice as strong as madak. The licensed places in the towns where opium was smoked were squalid and insanitary places. These were known as chandu-khaanas and were generally looked down upon. The then Chief Inspector of the Bombay Opium Department, Jehangir Rustom Pestonji published a book titled, *A Short History of the Lives of Bombay Opium Smokers*, which contained short biographies of 222 opium smokers.

The report of the Royal Commission formed the basis of British government policy, which stayed about the same till 1947. The views of the government are contained in the famous despatch of Lord Harding's Government in 1911, which had become as it were a *locus classicus* of the Government of India on the subject. It concluded, 'Whatever may be the case in other countries, centuries of inherited experience have taught the people of India discretion in the use of the drug, and its misuse is a negligible feature in Indian life.'

An Indian publication (Chopra, 1928) too noted, 'Be that as it may, there is no doubt that, in spite of its unrestricted availability and its low cost, the total consumption of opium in India was infinitely smaller than in China and other opium-using countries in the East. The percentage of habitual consumers was less than 1% of the total population except in the central districts of Punjab, populated chiefly by the Sikhs, where the consumption of opium recorded is perhaps the highest with the exceptions of Assam and Calcutta.' Assam in 1928 constituted all the current Northeastern states.

It is interesting to note that then as well as now, almost a hundred years later, not only does the number of 'habitual users' of opiates continue to be less than 1% of the population in India, but the Northeastern states and Punjab continue to be higher opioid consuming states of the country as found in a nationwide survey in 2019. What has changed, however, is the nature of preferred opioids from natural plant product opium to more harmful to semi-synthetic and synthetic products like heroin in the whole of the country.

Currently, India is one of the few countries in the world legally authorized to produce opium and the only country in the world to legally produce the resinous 'gum opium'. It is also the largest producer of legal opium in the world. Eleven other countries, i.e., Australia, Austria, France, China, Hungary, the Netherlands, Poland, Slovenia, Spain, Turkey and the Czech Republic cultivate opium poppy, but they do not extract gum. They cut the poppy bulb with eight inches of the stalk for processing in its entirety.

Almost at the same time as the Royal Opium Commission was set up, the British parliament also appointed a parallel Royal Hemp Commission to investigate the ill effects, if any, of the reported large-scale use of cannabis by Indians. The report of this Commission which ran into 3,281 pages, included testimonies from around 1,200 doctors, coolies, yogis, fakirs, heads of lunatic asylums, bhang peasants, tax gatherers, smugglers, army officers, hemp dealers, ganja palace operators and priests. According to the report, the Commission's visits to mental asylums all over India helped to negate the then prevailing belief that consumption of moderate amounts of ganja causes insanity.

~

Heroin was produced from morphine in the late 19th century. The 'problem' is the relative ease with which morphine can be extracted from opium and then heroin 'cooked' from morphine by a simple chemical process called acetylation. This case is the reason hundreds of 'kitchens' dot the two regions of the Golden Crescent and the Golden Triangle towards the west and the east of India. These two geographical regions produce most of the opium and traffic most of the heroin consumed in the world today. The Golden Crescent includes parts of Afghanistan, Iran and Pakistan and the mountainous peripheries of the area define the crescent. The Golden Triangle is the area where the borders of Thailand, Laos and Myanmar meet, and this area too is surrounded by hills. 'Kitchens' is a euphemism for makeshift, do-it-yourself laboratories which have sprung up in the hills and forests of these areas.

Today, Afghanistan is the number one and Myanmar the number two opium-producing country in the world. According to a UNODC report, a marked increase in opium poppy cultivation and a gradual increase in opium poppy yields in Afghanistan resulted in opium production in the country reaching 9,000 tons in 2017, an increase of 87% from the previous year. Among the drivers of that increase were political instability, lack of government control and reduced economic opportunities for rural communities, which may have left the rural population vulnerable to the influence of groups involved in the drug trade (UNODC, 2018).

Outside Asia, opium is also grown in Columbia and

Mexico. However, it is Afghanistan alone which produces 90% of the illegal opium in the world and supplies most of the heroin consumed by the world. Afghans themselves have used the poppy for millennia and even the clergy of the strictly Sunni country otherwise against all forms of intoxication rationalise growing opium thus: 'Opium is permissible because it is consumed by "kafirs" (infidels) of the West and not by Muslims or Afghans' (EFSAS, 2017). A 2010 survey on Drug Use in Afghanistan done by UNODC showed that around one million Afghans (aged 15-64) suffered from drug addiction. At 8% of the population, this rate is twice the global average.

From India's point of view, it is important to note that the distance between Amritsar and Afghanistan is a mere four hundred kilometres and those four hundred kilometres are Pakistani territory, a country whose security agencies, considering the visceral hostility between India and Pakistan, have no interest whatsoever in stopping the flow into Indian Punjab. In fact, it serves their purpose and aligns with the strategic interests of their deep state.

While the Punjab border has been the transit route for heroin and opium from Afghanistan through Pakistan to Delhi and onwards, in recent years, Punjab is being treated by the drug cartels not just as a transit point but as a destination consumer state in its own right. The Punjab police has been catching more smugglers bringing heroin into Punjab from Delhi rather than the other way around. In February 2020, the Special Task Force (STF) of Punjab charged with stopping narcotic smuggling, seized 188 kgs of heroin from a house in Amritsar. This huge cache had entered India not from the Pakistan border 30 kms away but from the Gujarat coast 1,500 kms away, and then transported all the way to Punjab.

CHAPTER 2

The Early Days, Natural Drugs and a More Tolerant Society

It is a myth that the people of Punjab have latched on to drugs only in recent years from previously having been ascetically abstinent. As mentioned in Chapter 1, an Indian publication in 1928 noted that the Northeastern states and Punjab have a higher proportion of people 'habitual' to opium than the rest of India. Punjabis have always had an inherently contradictory attitude towards intoxicants. A benign tolerance has existed in uncomfortable juxtaposition with the predominant religion Sikhism's censorious approach towards all intoxicants.

Excise on alcohol and drugs was a major source of revenue during Maharaja Ranjit Singh's rule despite a loose system of collection.

There were two rates of duties on liquor, one for the district of Lahore and the other for the rest of Punjab. In villages, there were no licensed monopolies for the sale of liquor, and anyone who wanted to could distil liquor in their own house without hindrance. No duty was levied for minor shops established for the sale of liquor but in large cities like Lahore, Amritsar and Jullundur, an annual fee had to be paid for distillation and sale.

The Sikh chiefs, however, could distil liquor in their own homes for themselves and their dependants and were not required to pay any duty.

Under the Sikh Empire, there were no separate fiscal arrangements regarding opium cultivation. However, higher rates of land tax were levied for cultivating opium as compared to other crops. The poppy plant was cultivated both in the hills and the plains of Punjab, but good opium could only be obtained in some parts of the hills. In the plains, the amount of opium found in poppy heads was less and these were mostly used as whole, either as decoction or smoked.

When the British annexed Punjab in 1849, the excise from drugs and alcohol saw a spurt thrice over not so much from an increase in consumption than the tightening of the system of collection, although popular lore was that the spread of English education had led to a loosening of morals and hence the increase in the rate of intoxication! The spirits were mostly a decoction of molasses but soon enough 'European liquor' was available in stores which was mostly cheap French brandy but also spirits manufactured at Murree (now in Pakistan) and rum made at Shahjahanpur.

Licenses to sell imported wines, liquors and beer, wholesale and retail, were granted at the following rates per annum (Kapur, 1931) in different categories of cities and towns:

1st Class — Rs 100
2nd Class — Rs 48
3rd Class — Rs 24
4th Class — Rs 6
5th Class — Rs 1

This classification of cities and towns was made to provide for places where demand was small, and shops would not have been opened if the fee had been high. Licenses to prepare malt liquor using the European method were granted free of charge. There was no duty on malt liquor but the brewer had to take out a wholesale license to sell beer.

Poppy cultivation under British rule, however, was placed under certain restrictions. The cultivator could grow enough for his own consumption, but all opium grown beyond that limit had to be sold to the government monopolist under penalties. The lease of the monopoly of retail sale of opium included the right to sell both Punjab-grown opium, and opium imported from other Indian States or from other countries. The lease also included the right to sell other drugs, the principal of which was charas, a strong cannabis product made from the resin of the plant, imported from Yarkand and Kabul. As far as bhang (the mildest version of intoxicant compared to ganja and charas made from the same plant) goes, it was difficult to regulate then as it is now since unlike the poppy plant, it grew wild in the hills and the adjacent plains and unlike charas, it did not require any skilled labour to prepare.

Most of central Punjab from Bahawalpur in the south to Ladakh in the north, including the cities of Lahore, Amritsar and Multan was called 'Bhangi Empire' in the 18th century because it was ruled by a *misl* (clan). Most of its members including the *misl* chief Sardar Chajja Singh and the soldiers regularly drank bhang which they served to guests too. (Dalbir Singh, 2010).

When the 'Bhangis' took over Lahore they came to possess the massive Zamzama cannon built earlier on the orders of the Afghan invader Ahmad Shah Durrani. It came to be known as Bhangian di Toap, a name it proudly retains today as it stands in the middle of Mall Road in Lahore outside the Lahore Museum. Rudyard Kipling, in his novel *Kim*, immortalized it in English literature as Kim's Gun.

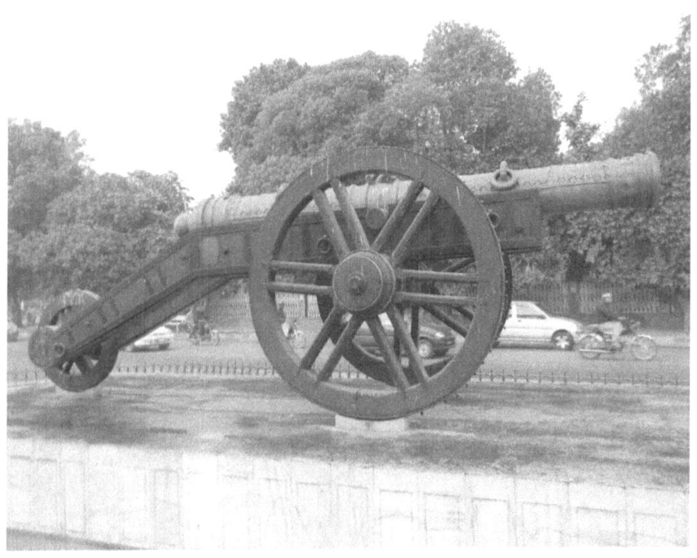

Bhangian di Toap, Mall Road, Lahore. (*Wikimedia Commons*)

Even today, Nihangs, a warrior sub-sect of Sikhism who are distinguishable in appearance by their unique long, blue martial dress, and pursue a semi-nomadic way of life take bhang regularly, which they prepare ritualistically on the Hola Mohalla festival. The usage is routine despite religious bans from mainstream Sikhism. The Nihangs call bhang *sukh-nidhan*—the giver of peace and happiness.

~

Although exact figures are available only for recent years, the tolerant attitude in Punjab towards alcohol and opium did not translate into large-scale runaway consumption. There are frequent references to *amlis* (addicts) and *postis* (people addicted to poppy husk) in early Punjabi literature and these are derogatory words. At the time of the Partition each village had a small number of people who took 'post' or drank regularly. On the other hand, celebratory drinking was quite another thing and enjoyed social approval then as now.

Of the hundreds of weddings I have been to, both in villages and cities in Punjab, there were very few where alcohol was not served. A nationwide survey found that 28.5 % of people in Punjab had one drink or more in the previous one year which put it at third place among Indian states after Tripura and Chhattisgarh (National Magnitude Survey, 2019). However, Punjab is not among the high per-capita alcohol consuming states in the country. Dadra and Nagar Haveli, Arunachal Pradesh, Andaman and Nicobar Islands, Andhra Pradesh, Telangana, Daman and Diu, Sikkim and Pondicherry rank higher (*Ambrosia*, 2021).

It is just the open, almost in-your-face way alcohol is consumed that gives Punjab its reputation. As you enter any marriage venue, the makeshift bar can be seen from the entrance. However, this is as much about a near-zero stigma as far as drinking is concerned as it is about conspicuous spending being a Punjabi trait.

In neighbouring Haryana, closely behind Punjab, with 21.5 % current users, it is not considered socially acceptable to be seen drinking openly even during weddings (except in Gurgaon and Faridabad which have more of a metropolitan than provincial character). I remember attending a wedding in Rohtak years back. Somebody came up to me and asked if I would like to have a drink. When I said, 'maybe', I was led up a staircase to a room on the terrace where some men were cloistered, drinking and smoking, while the main wedding went on merrily on the lawns below.

In Punjab, when a male toddler approaches his father in the evening, it is not uncommon for the latter to dip the tip of his finger in his glass and let the child suck it, feeling quite chuffed up in the process. 'Drinking is what the "Jutt" sons do,' is the patriarchal message.

In the National Magnitude Survey, Punjab found itself topping the dubious list of proportion of under eighteen persons having had one or more drink in the previous one year. This does not necessarily mean problem drinking in the future or even currently, but it certainly indicates the cavalier attitude towards alcohol and a scant regard for the legal age of drinking.

As far as the typical profile of regular opium users in Punjab till the late 80s is concerned, it was that of a well-functioning middle-aged farmer and the prevalence as judged from anecdotal evidence was moderate. Distinct from that was the specific and circumscribed common practice of giving farm workers opium husk during the backbreaking harvest season twice a year so that they would work tirelessly. This practice continues even now but to a lesser extent.

However, till the 90s, psychiatrists saw very few cases of opioid addiction in the clinics because whatever people were doing was not considered addiction by society, by families and certainly not by them, although from all accounts it certainly was. Psychiatrists sensed, when patients were brought in for a psychiatric disorder which had nothing to do with opium addiction, that addiction was a problem. Routinely filled proforma of the detailed psychiatric history of every patient included questions about intake of intoxicants and fairly common opium use in men was an incidental finding. The proforma also included questions about *family history* of addiction, if any. And a good number of large rural extended families, which was the norm then, had at least one male member who had been taking opium regularly for years. But even if that person was sitting in the doctor's clinic along with the patient, the psychiatrist could not have told him apart. And nobody else could have either. Punjab was then a state with a good number of high-functioning opium addicts. This was hardly a secret since there was no stigma involved.

Out of the people who took intoxicants, the middle classes and the well to do in the villages took pure opium, which came in the form of a dark gum; the poor in the villages took poppy husk as a light, coarse powder, brownish in colour, which was bulky but if taken in sufficient quantity over the course of the day delivered the same amount of opium to the user. The city people drank and that was all there was to it. The vast majority of people, of course, then as now, neither drank nor took any other intoxicant.

As a young psychiatrist, I was often called by surgeon colleagues to other city hospitals or the ones in nearby towns to see patients admitted for routine surgeries when at the last moment it was discovered that the patient was an opium addict and the surgery was held up for this reason. The standard advice by all psychiatrists in such situations was this: let the patient take his usual dose the evening before the surgery and half the daily dose after the surgery as soon as he was conscious. On subsequent days he was to go back to whatever amount he had been taking earlier. And of course, the anaesthetist must be told about the opium habit. Medical practitioners in Punjab had devised a safe way to work around and manage the patient's opium habit as a part of treating the whole patient.

This steered clear of reckless measures to stop the drug intake, treat the withdrawal which would have taken days or weeks and shifted the focus away from the hernia or the hip surgery, which the patient had actually come for. What helped enormously was the medical evidence that pure opium unlike alcohol, even when taken for decades, rarely caused any organ damage or metabolic disturbance. And the relative cultural tolerance of opium took care of the morality aspect.

Since opium addiction was not seen as a problem, least of all by the patient himself, very few men came for treatment just to get rid of opium. And remember, this was Punjab, today considered by many as a state so destabilized by opioid addiction that movies are being made on it and elections won and lost over it.

I had been in psychiatry for three years when I laid eyes on my first patient of opium addiction, who approached the department of psychiatry specifically for treatment of his addiction. His name was Surjeet Singh. He was a tall, lanky, turbanned farmer with a flowing beard. He always wore a long kurta pyjama, over which across the front and back there would be prominently visible, the diagonal strap of his kirpan. Surjeet was sixty, a widower and he lived with some farmhands. He had been elected village sarpanch for several terms consecutively and was known as a cool-headed and wise man to whom farmers from nearby villages came for advice and arbitration in land disputes.

He told me he had been taking a small amount of opium every day for over thirty years but now he wanted to get rid of it. I explained to him that this would need admission. It was the late 70s and we did not have very effective drugs to smoothen opiate withdrawal. The treatment used to be a rocky, uncomfortable and painful affair lasting for three or four weeks. And there was no guarantee that mild aches and pains, not to mention craving, would not persist long after discharge. I was curious to know why he wanted to leave opium. His dose was small: one *tola* which is ten grams, lasted him a week. It had not caused him any harm so far and was not likely to in the future.

His motive was unusual. His only offspring, a son who

drove a city bus in Vancouver, had got married to an Irish girl, a waitress, two years ago. The wedding happened before a registrar and there was no time for Surjeet to apply for a visa. But the following winter, the couple had come to Punjab and stayed with him in the village house. Surjeet, a taciturn man himself, liked his high-spirited daughter-in-law who was a first-generation immigrant from a farming family in an Irish village. The couple had a son the previous year. After going back, Surjeet's son had applied for a resident visa for his father, which had now come through.

'So, I want to get rid of opium because I would not get it in Canada, and my daughter-in-law does not even know that I take it.' he explained.

Surjeet braved the treatment and went to Canada, opium free as he wanted. There were several others like him that I treated in the subsequent years. But the inflow of patients looking for treatment before immigrating to Canada stopped in the following decades. When I asked a farmer friend the possible reason for it, he replied, 'Because now opium is available in Canada too!'

The only addiction that psychiatrists treated those days was alcoholism, and a smattering of patients addicted to short acting barbiturates—Seconal (Secobarbital) being a common brand. Since barbiturates are strong drugs, these were also a common method of suicide in the 60s and 70s, being handy, painless and having gained a touch of dark glamour after Marilyn Monroe reportedly killed herself with an overdose.

If from the above narratives you get the impression that everybody in the 70s, 80s and 90s had a pragmatic and rational attitude towards all addictions, let me disabuse you of the notion. Opium addiction, although not very prevalent, was the one best tolerated by society because most people who took opium by and large functioned normally. Other addictions were frowned upon. Cannabis addiction, on the social approval hierarchy of addictions, was at the lowest rung. This was because cannabis or charas addiction is often synonymous with sloth and laziness. The belief is probably without any basis.

While drinking was tolerated and even considered manly, getting drunk and needing help were disapproved of. Men lying on the roadside and smelling of alcohol were and still are left alone out of contempt. This is tragic because some of those men may be diabetics and may have had just a drink or two, which in turn leads to low blood sugar levels and unconsciousness. All of this is treatable if the patient is taken to a hospital in time but if left untreated, it can be fatal. All other addictions—particularly those involving tablets or injections—were highly stigmatized.

Let me share the story of a patient whom I treated for barbiturate addiction and shouldn't have. The patient herself was certainly less than keen to be treated.

It was one of those drizzly, freezing days in the last week of December which Chandigarh specialises in. Since it was the winter break many resident doctors had gone home. I was manning the post-lunch OPD alone. The OPD was deserted. I clearly remember the young girl, Sherry, even after all these years. She peeped into my cabin wearing a long jacket and carrying a mineral water bottle. Mineral water bottles in those days meant just one thing—a foreigner. Coming straight to the point, she told me she was a student from Canada who was visiting relatives during the Christmas holidays.

She was a barbiturate addict and her supply of Seconal tablets had been confiscated from her bag by customs officials at Delhi airport. A few tablets were left in her pocket and she had consumed those. She had not had Seconal for the last twenty-four hours, had not slept the previous night and her taut expression was interrupted by twitches. I sensed she could already be in early withdrawal. She sheepishly asked if she could get a prescription for just enough tablets to last her for the remaining ten days of her trip. She had already been to the hospital pharmacy and found out that they had Seconal. A prescription was all that she needed.

And I could have written one for her. There was no law against it. Those days, it was prescribed for insomnia which she was certainly having. Had I done that, she would have settled down quickly and gone back to the village near Morinda she was visiting. At the end of the trip, she would have returned to the part of the globe she had come from, and nothing would have been amiss.

But I did not do that because there was this fuzzy notion in my mind that providing drugs to addicts is not what doctors do. If she had lied and complained only of insomnia, without mentioning addiction, I would have prescribed Seconal without a qualm. I was quite junior at that time and there was nobody available for me to consult. Still, nothing excuses the most illogical, impractical and wasteful treatment process available under the circumstances that I set in motion

Barbiturate withdrawal is a medical emergency requiring admission since it can cause non-stop epileptic fits, a condition called 'status epilepticus'. So, I made her call the family with whom she was staying and admitted her to the ward after they consented on the phone since she herself was just seventeen. By doing so I unleashed a chain of events, which in hindsight, I know were disruptive and unnecessary. Sherry stayed in the hospital for four weeks thus missing Christmas, New Year and her classes. And a team of doctors including me treated her with the same class of drugs that she was addicted to, and gradually reduced the dose. She had to postpone her return flight by six weeks, which in those days was a cumbersome and exorbitant process.

Far more catastrophically, the relatives whom she had come to visit looking for her roots, came to know that the charming niece of theirs in faded jeans and boots, who had become a favourite of the extended clan in just a day, was a drug addict so badly affected that she needed to be admitted to a psychiatry ward. And of course, the girl's parents in Canada who might have had their suspicions but were not sure about her drug habit came to know of it too. They dropped everything to fly to India to be with her. This whole exercise was carried out while the patient kept saying that she was not ready yet, that she had insecurities and hurts which made her resort to drugs and she was not willing to talk to anyone about them. She was in India for a very short while and in any case, she did not trust us. She swore she would go back to her addiction the moment she landed in her Toronto neighbourhood, which I came to know later, she did.

Half a century later, as far as treatment of addictions is concerned, society continues to by and large do what I did then—inject our personal and borrowed morality into the scientific concept of treatment of addictions.

~

In the late 80s, psychiatrists in Punjab started to see patients of drug addiction in their clinics in significant numbers, a trickle at first, it soon became a continuous flow. But these were not the usual heavy drinkers in their forties with liver problems or the moderately rich middle-aged farmers taking opium or even the poorer farmhands addicted to the bulkier *bhukki.*

Something was changing and changing fast. For one, addicts were becoming younger. Frightfully younger. Drugs were changing too. Those who were showing up at clinics were young men addicted to synthetic opioids like capsules of Dextropropoxyphene nicknamed 'proxy', which was then commonly used as a pain reliever by surgeons and orthopaedic doctors for their trauma and post-surgery patients. The young men who were misusing these would buy them over the counter from chemists who were happy to oblige. Chemists' shops had sprouted all over Punjab like mushrooms after a spell of rain and they were fully licensed by the government. They were of course required to sell these drugs only on prescription and keep a record, both of which they did not do.

When questioned by the press, the government pleaded a shortage of drug inspectors. Chemists' shops were located in the cities, small towns and even on the narrow link roads which criss-cross the whole state. Even in remote places where you could not find a mechanic for miles if your scooter broke down, you could find a licensed chemist's shop to buy enough capsules of proxy to keep you high for a month. Nobody has ever asked the Punjab government why thousands of licenses for chemists' shops were given when it was clear that the only way those many shops could have stayed afloat was by selling habit-forming medicines over the counter.

Opiates have been justifiably used for thousands of years as a highly effective treatment for cough and diarrhoea. Codeine, a natural opiate and a component of opium, has been a legitimate component of popular cough syrups like Corex for decades. Similarly, tablets of Diphenoxylate (brand name Lomotil), a synthetic opioid, has been used as an emergency drug to stop severe diarrhoea. All three drugs have an opium-like effect if taken in high doses. And the amounts ingested by these young men were very high. Two hundred tablets of Lomotil or forty capsules of Proxyvon, or ten bottles of hundred millilitre Corex syrup a day were the average intake by patients who were now coming to the clinics. And in many cases, instead of this OR that, it was this AND that.

That was the time when people setting out on morning walks started finding parks in the cities and towns of Punjab littered with empty bottles of cough syrup and used strips of proxy capsules, and the parents of young men began panicking at the sight of empty bottles found in the vicinity of their houses.

A notable feature of the case histories as recorded in psychiatric clinics at that time was the occupation of the young patients. It often went like this:

'What does he do?'

Parent: 'Nothing.'

'What was he doing earlier?'

'Nothing.'

If one probed further into the history of the patient the following would come to light: he was in school, an average enough student, a bit stubborn and quarrelsome but that profile fit in with the overall average at that age. He had then joined a college in a nearby town, either a degree course in humanities or more commonly a diploma in hospitality or in management. Bachelor in Business Administration (BBA) was a course commonly offered. Why? Because the parents were told this was a job-oriented course and at two lakh rupees, admission was cheap. And there were chances of going abroad, as the father would report. And why would he need a job? The family had land, nobody in the family had taken up a job before. The boy did not want to do farming because over the previous three generations, three brothers had had nine grandsons—forget the daughters because they are not counted in Punjab or anywhere else for that matter in North India for the purpose of inheritance. And the family's twenty acres had become two over three generations.

All along there had been indications of a change in behaviour which were attributed by indulgent families to the misguided adage: 'boys will be boys'. They had been coming home late, sleeping till very late, spending too much money on 'god knows what' as far as their mothers knew. The mothers were the ones who were more amenable to cajoling, coaxing, manipulation and threats of self-harm. Their sons cooked up excuses: 'We need money for petrol, my motorcycle needs repair, it is a friend's birthday and everybody is bringing presents, there is a new movie playing at the theatre and all the boys are going.' The rude awakening would come when there was a fight or an accident under the effect of intoxicants or sometimes a frightening seizure when the young man happened to take more proxy capsules than usual. There were variations in the story like a romantic breakup which the desperate parents latched on to as the cause. But the fact that did not change was that the young man did nothing either then or later. And the breakup was often the result rather than the cause of addiction.

A study conducted at the Medical College, Faridkot in central Punjab and published in the *Indian Journal of Psychiatry* reported that between 1994 and 1998, the use of opium decreased in Punjab by approximately 40% while the use of the cheap substitute, poppy husk, increased by 55%. Over and above this the use of pharmaceutical opiates like proxy, Corex and Lomotil by youngsters, which were even cheaper and easily available doubled (Sachdeva et al, 2002). This simple observation was fraught with significance for anybody who observed the field of drug addiction in Punjab because behind those ordinary figures lay the lengthening shadow of social and economic changes plaguing the state, a slippery slope that has not levelled off till today.

A short sketch of the chronology of opioid intake in Punjab would be approximately go like this, with a lot of overlapping and sub-regional variations:

Before 1985: Natural opioids. Mostly opium but also opium husk colloquially called *bhukki* or *dode*—the poor man's opium, cheap but bulkier quantities needed to be taken for same degree of effect. Supply of opium was from Afghanistan and Rajasthan and that of husk from Rajasthan where it was legally grown and available to people with addiction on permits.

1985-2000: The ratio starts changing in favour of cheaper husk and pharmaceutical opioids like Proxyvon, Corex and Lomotil.

2000-07: Pharmaceutical opioids predominate and also the demography of opioid addicts changes from men predominantly aged thirty to fifty years to younger men in their twenties.

2007-2012: Heroin, both the street form called smack and the pure form called *chitta* becomes the predominant opioid addiction in Punjab gradually phasing out pharmaceutical opioids as the government belatedly comes down hard on chemists.

Present: Heroin continues to be the most common opioid used by 80-90% of people with opioid addiction in Punjab.

The reason which drove this change from natural to semi-synthetic and synthetic opioids, not just in Punjab, but eventually all over India and many other countries, lay in America and its so-called War on Drugs. This 'war' enforced total prohibition of all drugs including opioids across the world through international treaties sponsored by the West. The most visible and also the most harmful effect of prohibition is that it converts the intoxicants that are available to people from *milder and bulkier* to *stronger and concentrated* because the latter are less likely to be detected in transit and hence easier to smuggle.

That is why whenever and wherever there is prohibition of alcohol in the world, the only alcoholic beverages that are available are those with high alcohol content like whiskey, gin and vodka. Smugglers find it difficult and riskier to smuggle in beer and beer drinkers are thus coaxed into drinking whiskey or vodka available in the alleys, if they want to have that weekend drink. The conundrum of prohibition comes from the simple fact that it is easier to smuggle a van filled with whiskey bottles than a truck full of beer bottles into a state with prohibition.

While the international treaties that India was signatory to banned the production, trade and *even use* of all drugs obtained directly from any of the three plants—opium, cannabis and coca and their chemical analogues, Indian delegates to these UN conventions, to their credit, managed to salvage bhang from being banned citing traditional and cultural reasons and the fact that bhang is commonly used during religious festivals. How bhang was exempted as a concession to countries like India is in itself interesting. Without mentioning bhang, the Single Convention on Narcotic Drugs, 1961, defined cannabis as follows:

'Cannabis means the flowering or fruiting tops of the cannabis plant (excluding the seeds and leaves when not accompanied by the tops) from which the resin has not been extracted.' Cannabis, thus defined, was what was banned by the UN convention. Since bhang is prepared from the leaves of the same plant, it was not banned, while ganja or marijuana, which are extracted from the flowering tops were. As was charas which comes from the resin.

This could have been a good way for India to promote a mild and internationally legal intoxicant, which could have been easily regulated and sold in government or private stores. Most Indian states, however, took the moral path and did not make use of the pragmatic concession which its experts had managed to extract from the international community, to provide a mild, cheap, relatively safe, and some would even say, the safest intoxicant, to people.

While most states neither banned the consumption nor allowed the sale of bhang, states like Bihar and Assam prohibited it through specific legislations. Bihar did it through the Bihar Prohibition and Excise Act, 2016, which made sale and use of both alcohol and all products of cannabis, *including* bhang, illegal and prosecutable. In Assam the Ganja and Bhang Prohibition Act, 1958, prohibits the sale, purchase, possession and consumption of both ganja and bhang.

At present, the states of UP, MP, Rajasthan, Orissa and Chhattisgarh regulate the sale of bhang through licensed outlets. Bhang is popular in holy cities like Varanasi because according to some, Brahmins, the holy class, are not allowed to consume alcohol or tobacco leaving bhang as the only option for them. And bhang according to Hindu religious belief comes with the blessings of Bhole Shankar, Lord Shiva.

To make the situation about cannabis even more nuanced, it is worth mentioning that in Punjab, the cannabis plant grows wild although connoisseurs would scoff at the quality. The state government even makes some money out of it. Every year, for the last thirty years, it has been auctioning the rights to harvest this plant growing on the roadside to a lone bhang vend in district Hoshiarpur (*The Times of India*, May 13, 2014). The contractor, Wadia Group, even paid Rs 8.8 lakh to the Punjab government as VAT for the year 2013-14 according to excise records. It sold the produce to Rajasthan and Madhya Pradesh since the Punjab government does not allow it to be sold in the state. Although there would have been no legal hindrance as per national laws or international treaties, if the Punjab government had wanted to. Once again, morality rather than logic prevailed.

CHAPTER 3

Punjab: Green Revolution Backtracking, Addictions as Partial Suicides

I met Narinder Kaur one August afternoon, when, despite the rain and the slush on the roads, her distraught husband brought her to my clinic on his motorcycle, all the way from their village located on the Doraha canal. She was in her early fifties and was having what appeared to be a panic attack. Her husband said she had never suffered from anything like this before. Her face was frozen with anxiety, her body so tremulous she had to be supported and she could not breathe easily. Talking clearly required effort on her part.

Her husband had no idea what was happening; the village GP had told them it appeared to be a psychological problem and had sent them to me. After I sent the husband out of the room, gave her a glass of water, and an anti-anxiety tablet to keep under her tongue, she settled down quickly. When I asked her if something specific had triggered the attack, she fished out a tiny polythene pouch filled with a brownish white powder from her *kameez* (loose tunic) pocket.

To me, it became clear what had happened. Narinder was yet another mother in Punjab who had discovered street heroin while emptying her son's pockets before doing the laundry.

Mothers with young sons learnt from newspapers and television reports what a pouch of heroin looked like and prayed they never would have to see one in real life. She had not yet confided in her husband because he had unstable blood pressure and although she strongly suspected the white powder was what she feared, she was not completely sure yet. She told me later that there had been signs in her son's behaviour all along that she failed to recognise. After spending half-a-day in the clinic, Narinder went home symptom-free and the focus shifted to her son Navjot, who was brought to the clinic the next morning.

Navjot, I was told, had initially refused to come. When his father confronted him with the pouch of heroin, he had shot back, 'So what? You drink half a bottle of liquor every day, don't you? I take this.' After the outburst he had clung to his mother, cried, and apologized to his father and confessed he had started snorting smack six months back after he failed the IELTS examination. IELTS is the standard English examination those who want to go abroad on a study or immigration visa to English-speaking countries are required to take.

I had heard a lot about IELTS from my young patients, a good number of whom aspired to go to North America or the UK or Australia. In the past twenty years, on my way to work I have noticed that an IELTS coaching course is the most advertized product on the walls of the city, and this is true for the whole state of Punjab. The only large hoardings which have survived the economic slowdown are those of the IELTS coaching centres. It is difficult to find a young man/woman who does not want to go abroad for good. Narinder and her husband went on to reiterate before me what I had been hearing for years from other rural families.

Navjot's grandfather owned thirty acres of land and theirs was a relatively prosperous family in not just their own village but even in the surrounding villages too. Navjot's father had three brothers and each inherited seven-and-a-half acres. His father and his elder brother farmed that land but the holding being small, it was barely cost effective. If Navjot wanted to do farming like every adult male in the family so far, he and his brother would have less than four acres each after their father passed away. Hence, the family's plan for him to get a college degree and go to Canada made sense. In Scarborough, Canada, Narinder's nephew was part owner of a petrol pump. Navjot could work at the pump till he got a better job. To pay for Navjot's college admission and the advance the travel agent demanded, one acre of land in the small town across the canal was mortgaged to an *arhtia*, a commission agent, whom the family sold their farm produce to twice a year.

But as of then, both the university degree and the visa seemed to be beyond reach. As Navjot told his parents, even though he did get ready and leave the house every morning on his motorcycle to go to the university there was really no university to go to. He had been suspended for six months after a fight with another student a while ago. He was intoxicated when he had picked the fight. He had kept the expulsion a secret from his parents. Even before that he had been irritable for months, sleeping late and waking up late, dressing sloppily which alone should have made the parents suspicious, since he had been a rather natty dresser before.

That was three years back. Navjot was in and out of heroin addiction for the next two years but after he got a job, he has been clean for over a year. He could not go to Canada because although he did get a degree eventually, that degree was not recognized in Canada. He now works as a salesman at a shopping mall that has sprung up outside the city. He commutes from his village forty-five minutes each way daily because his salary is not enough for him to rent a room in the city. But the job has certainly been a turning point. The mooring of a routine and socialising with friends from work, including a young woman from the neighbouring village he has been seeing, have been crucial in keeping him out of trouble so far. As the saying goes, 'the opposite of addiction is not sobriety but human connection.'

Equally vital is the treatment that has been continuing for three years although there were interruptions caused by relapses during the first two years. Navjot comes in for counselling and medication once in two weeks and makes it a point to say hello to me whenever he is here. He has even referred other patients, young men like him, to me.

Narinder never had a second panic attack and has been the emotional bulwark for her son. This is the main reason things have not been as bad with Navjot as they often are with other young men in a similar situation. Relatively speaking, Navjot's is one of the feel-good stories. Most are not.

~

Any schoolboy will tell you that the capital of Punjab is Chandigarh but the truth is far more nuanced. Chandigarh is also the capital of the neighbouring state of Haryana while Chandigarh is neither in Punjab nor in Haryana, but a union territory governed by the central government. The capital of Punjab is outside Punjab! This freak arrangement has worked exceedingly well for the politicians and bureaucrats of Punjab. They get to live in a modern city as VIP guests without the headache of governing it. Chandigarh has some of the best colleges and the most advanced health care facilities in India, not to mention beautiful golf courses, a modern airport and three Shatabdi Expresses plying to Delhi in a day. Ironically, till

2011, Chandigarh had no rail connection to Punjab of which it is the capital. Unsurprisingly, hardly any senior politicians or senior officials of the Punjab government settle down in Punjab after retirement. Padma Bhushan Dr S.S. Johl is a rare exception. He is the seniormost agricultural economist of the country, a former vice-chancellor of Punjab Agricultural University and of Punjab University, former chairperson of the Agriculture Price Commission of India, director of the Central Board of Governors of the Reserve Bank of India, consultant to the World Bank and Food & Agricultural Organization of UNO and the current chancellor of Punjab Central University.

Ninety-two-year-old Dr Johl talked to me on a winter morning, sitting in the sun-swept veranda of his modest house in Ludhiana. We discussed the golden days of farming in Punjab, what went wrong, the connections between the Green Revolution backtracking and addictions, and how it can all still be turned around.

After independence, when India chalked out its first five year plan in 1950-51, the country found itself facing a dire shortage of food grains because of very low yield of both wheat and rice per acre in the whole country. This situation was not going to rectify itself anytime in the foreseeable future. It is not a well-known fact any longer (nor does anybody want to be reminded of it) that in 1961, India was on the brink of a mass famine and was living on one wheat-laden ship from the USA to the next. The USA was producing surplus wheat then and that surplus was exported to several food-deficient countries including India. Since these countries did not have foreign exchange reserves to pay for the wheat, they were magnanimously allowed by the USA to pay in their own currencies.

Indian media called it PL-480 wheat, and many believed it was the name of a specific variety. PL-480, in fact, was short for

Public Law-480, an American bill signed by President Eisenhower in 1954. The programme managed to stabilise wheat prices in the USA which had plunged, demand being less than supply. The programme simultaneously created secondary markets in the world for American agricultural produce and promoted international trade in general in favour of the USA. Over and above that, there were large-scale foreign policy benefits for America, which such a major act of generosity brings with it for the donor country.

The USA spent the money paid for the wheat in developing countries from where it came, as per the agreement, but only in areas decided by the American government. Naturally, the USA spent it wherever it furthered American diplomatic interests. The arrangement however was grossly insufficient, extremely stretched out and could not have lasted for long. Dr Norman Borlaug, the renowned agricultural scientist who would later receive a Nobel Peace Prize for his work on developing high-yield, disease-resistant wheat varieties, was invited to India and a gargantuan project to pull the country permanently out of famine was initiated. This project which went on to be a memorable success would be called the Green Revolution.

In India, Punjab which included Haryana and parts of Himachal Pradesh at that time, was selected to be the first state to try the new high-yield seeds because of reliable water supply for irrigation from a network of canals constructed by the British. Punjab was also the only state where land consolidation had already happened by then. In other states, the farmers' small pieces of land were scattered around, making mechanized farming impractical. Other crucial factors were the availability of a hard-working populace experienced in farming, ample sunlight necessary for photosynthesis and a flat tabletop landscape.

The Green Revolution strategy succeeded in Punjab beyond

the wildest expectations with production of grains increasing several times, especially that of wheat and rice. A country plagued by chronic semi-famine became food surplus in a couple of years. The support by the central government by way of institutional mechanisms to ensure purchase of wheat and paddy at an assured minimum support price or MSP made all the difference. The system was both technology intensive and manpower intensive, the latter more so during harvesting seasons twice a year.

All of this happened because of the forward-looking entrepreneurial skills of Punjabis who were ready to take risks in trying out new methods. Another factor was the presence of a very large number of serving and retired army men in Punjab, which ensured a minimum educational qualification and a comfort level in handling machinery of varying degrees of complexity and a willingness to experiment with those.

These initiatives made the rural economy of Punjab a model of economic development and prosperity. Labels like 'granary of India' and 'India's bread-basket' came in thick and fast. However, the new model was technology intensive and needed tractors, harvesters and other equipment. That required capital. Loans were available through banks owned by co-operative societies, but farmers were more comfortable with the *arhtias* with whom families had dealt for generations and who asked for very little paperwork. Soon, Punjab became the richest state in India with the highest per-capita income in the country. The boom lasted for over three decades.

Over successive generations, with the breaking up of large joint families even in villages, land holdings became smaller till the size of the farms stopped being cost-effective for technology-driven farming. The average farm size in Punjab at present is eight acres and only one-third of farms are over twenty acres.

The water table went down every year mainly because paddy is a water-guzzling crop and while canals in the areas provided a basic level of irrigation, the large quantity of extra water required during sowing and transplanting of paddy had to be pumped out from the earth. Traditional tube wells no longer worked because of the dip in the water table. This required the powerful submersible pumps to be sunk in deeper and deeper, which was costly and required credit. The electric supply in rural areas was erratic and so diesel motors had to be used, making the process even costlier.

In their anxiety to maximise yield, farmers used more fertilisers which decreased the fertility of soil and polluted the water over the years. Theoretically, industrial infrastructure is supposed to take over from an agricultural revolution after the latter has sustained a society for a fixed period. This is what happened in large parts of America, Europe and Asia and in many Indian states, including Punjab's neighbour Haryana. The so-called Green Revolution on the scale of a revolution was not expected to last forever by any account. As predicted by experts the gains plateaued in the early 80s, started to decline in the 90s and by the first decade of the millennium the party was over. In Punjab unlike elsewhere in India and in the world, there was no industrial backup to buffer the decline. Since it is a border state, which had borne the brunt of two vicious wars with Pakistan in 1965 and 1971, Indian industrialists had mostly stayed away from investing here.

Whatever little industry was already there fled during the decade-and-a-half of the violent, armed insurgency that gripped the state during the 80s and the early 90s. To make matters worse the central government offered tax benefits for starting new industries in the neighbouring state of Himachal Pradesh and as a result, many factories from Punjab shifted there.

Meanwhile, the small farmers became marginal and the marginal farmers became labourers in nearby grain markets or took on other jobs. These were early signs of a process of 'de-peasantisation' which continues today. My patient Navjot was just one among the hundreds of thousands who were extruded from farming and suffered terribly since the backup safety net of the industrial sector was missing.

~

In the late 80s, I was at a psychiatry conference in Bombay. In the darkened hall, I put up my first transparency (remember transparencies?), which was supposed to show among other things that Punjab was the number one state in India on per-capita income rankings and still had a fairly high incidence of mental illness. A colleague from Bombay pointed out that a correction was needed since Punjab no longer held the number one position. Maharashtra was at that position according to a recent ranking. He was right. That downward slide has continued over the years and today, Punjab is number nineteen among twenty-nine Indian states on per-capita income ranking. In 2021, the per-capita income in Punjab slid below the national average for the first time.

The subsequent years of globalization and privatization brought to the state, among other things, a rash of private universities. Punjab got more than its fair share for its small size. These universities charge exorbitant fees and do not refuse admission to anybody. Any student who stays long enough gets a diploma or a degree.

Punjab by then had a large number of youngsters belonging to rural families, who either did not have a family farm to run or very often did not want to join their fathers in farming because it was too much hard work for too little money. Many of them joined these new colleges and so-called deemed universities located in glossy buildings. In many instances, families like Navjot's mortgaged or sold a piece of land to admit their sons or daughters to these courses. Many of these degrees are not worth the paper they are printed on because whatever is taught and learned is not skill-oriented and there is no match with what the job market requires. All that these teaching shops do is substitute a large number of under-educated, unemployed youth in Punjab with educated, unemployable youth at a considerable cost to families.

The state was like a rich man who had become a pauper overnight. The people of Punjab, particularly the villagers, collectively as well as individually faced a situation where the old norms of life were no longer possible. And society was still struggling to put in place new norms and social support, leaving individuals rudderless. It was not just about money; it was equally about normlessness.

French sociologist Emile Durkheim wrote about the concept of 'anomie' in the late 19th century. It is a state of normlessness caused by a sudden change in the level of the individual's integration into society. The word comes from the Greek 'anomy', which means lawlessness except that this is not the lawlessness of the law-and-order type but of the rudderlessness variety. Durkheim called 'anomie' a state where the expectations of behaviour from individuals in a radically changed environment are unclear, and the support of the social system is weakening.

A few years later, Durkheim published, 'Le Suicide' which is considered a pathbreaking study of suicide. The principles of this work are applicable anywhere in the world at any given time. He described four types of suicide, one of which was 'anomic'. It 'happens in times of social and economic upheaval. People are unaware where they fit in within their societies. They do not know the limits on their desires and are constantly in a state of disappointment, because they follow the old norms when they were better off.' This type of suicide is due to the breakdown of equilibrium with society and can happen in contrasting situations; after sudden penury or suddenly becoming rich. In other words, anomic suicide takes place in a situation, which has cropped up more or less suddenly and unexpectedly.

While farmers' suicides have been a subject of intense discussion all over the country as a blazing sign of agrarian distress, surprisingly in Punjab, where it all started, the situation played out differently. While widespread agrarian distress is a hard economic reality visible to all in Punjab, there is no evidence that farmers as a group are proportionately overrepresented among those who commit suicide. This is surprising because in Punjab, the epicentre of farming distress, the rates of farmers' suicides were expected to be the highest in the country. But while the agricultural crisis causes immense mental distress and leaves the sufferers looking for a lifeline, the number of farmers' suicide in Punjab is statistically not more than in other occupations.

Part of the reason may be that suicide figures in general in Punjab have always been quite low as compared to the rest of the country. Suicide rates are expressed internationally as a number per hundred thousand of population per year. According to the National Crime Research Bureau, the suicide rate in India was 12.0 while for Punjab it was 8.5 in 2021.

Even while the state government gives monetary relief to the families of victims in cases of farmers' suicides (including families of farm hands), according to data sourced by *The Indian Express* from the Punjab Agriculture Department and Punjab Revenue Department, the Punjab government received information about only 2,528 such cases in the four years between 2015-18.

However, suicide can also be a matter of degree of self-harm and completed suicide may be just the extreme end of a spectrum of self-destructive behaviours. Karl Menninger, a leading psychoanalyst, considered drug addictions and alcoholism as partial suicides or chronic suicides implying similar underlying psychological mechanisms in suicides and drug addictions with self-destruction as the common theme (Colt, 1991).

If we look at human history closely to find the periods when addiction peaked dramatically, we can see that these were the times of such normlessness during which the lines to follow had been erased and community support had crumbled:

i) The native Americans of North America who were stripped of their land and culture by the white immigrants had lapsed into mass alcoholism.

ii) The English poor in early 18th-century Britain were driven out from their villages to far-off, scattered cities to work in factories. They responded by heavy drinking on a massive scale during afterhours to start with, but soon the distinction was lost. This wave of mass drinking was called 'gin-craze' as men and women were found drunk and lay sprawled on the streets and children were left uncared for. A series of five major Acts were passed by the British parliament between 1729-51 to control consumption of alcohol as the gin-craze reached its peak.

iii) In the 1970s and 80s, people in American inner cities were stripped of their factory jobs leading to a crack cocaine addiction epidemic (Dunlap et al, 2006).

As many of us glean from the posters put out by well-meaning NGOs, which work in this extremely challenging area, the primary factor in drug addiction is supposed to be the

DRUG. Hence the slogan, 'Just Say No (To Drugs)', the origin of which is ascribed to an early 80s campaign in the USA led by then first lady Nancy Reagan. The implication here is that there are some drugs so addictive that if you use any one a few times, it changes your brain in such a manner that you cannot live without the drug. It hijacks your brain in a manner of speaking. So, best is to say 'no' to drugs and nothing else would be required for you to stay drug-free. This belief also lays the entire blame on the supply side, implying that if societies could just stop the availability of drugs, all will be well. It is presumed that if drugs are lying around, most people will take them and get addicted.

However, the lesson learnt from the examples from recent history listed above, is that social and economic factors are more important than the availability/non-availability dimension. An interesting, rewarding and challenging social milieu in which the individual is connected to and supported by society is the most effective inoculation against addiction. Strong evidence for this line of thinking came from the field of animal experiments.

A striking advertisement that was aired on American television in the 70s explained it clearly. The commercial showed a rat in close-up licking a tiny bottle as the narrator said, 'Only one drug is so addictive, nine out of ten laboratory rats will use it. And use it. And use it. Until dead. It is called cocaine and it will do the same thing to you.' The rat ran around like a maniac and then, as promised, dropped dead while scary music played in the background. Similar experiments were done on rats to prove the addictiveness of heroin and other drugs. However, in all these experiments, the laboratory conditions were such that the rats lived one in each cage, and could neither see nor touch each other because the sides of their cages were made of sheet metal.

In the late 70s, Bruce Alexander, professor of experimental psychology in Canada, noticed that each rat was all alone with no sensory stimulation, no activities and no friends. There was nothing for it to do but to take drugs. Alexander decided to run the experiment differently. With the help of his team, he built two sets of homes for the laboratory rats (Alexander et al, 1981).

One set was like in the original experiment—a series of empty cages isolated from one another with one rat in each cage as if in solitary confinement with nothing to do except to get a fix. The other set of homes was like a paradise for rats. It contained nearly everything a rat could ever want; wheels and balls of all colours, the best rat food and other rats to hang out with and have sex with. Alexander called it 'Rat Park'. In this experiment, each set of rats had access to two drinking bottles. One contained plain water and the other morphine, a drug just like heroin. In the evening, both bottles in each set of homes were weighed to measure how much of each liquid had been consumed.

It was found that rats in the isolated cages consumed five times more morphine than the rats in the Rat Park. While even the latter had a 24x7 supply of morphine they, by and large, stayed sober. They chose to spend their time doing other interesting things, simply because there were other interesting things available to do. While follow-up studies have not shown results as dramatic as Alexander's original work, the Rat Park study was seminal in drawing attention to social factors in causation of addiction. Several subsequent studies have reinforced the effect of environmental enrichment on self-administration, such as one that showed environmental enrichment reduced re-instatement of cocaine-seeking behaviour in mice, even more so when the self-administration was mainly the result of stress and environmental cues (Chauvet et al, 2009; Solinas et al, 2009).

Punjab after the late 80s was certainly no Rat Park. The unemployment rate in rural youth had reached 16% and that did not include the very large number of under-employed. Something had to give. Left with almost nothing to do, it would have been surprising if drug addiction had not peaked dangerously and acquired such a destructive form among the young men of that and successive generations. To make things even worse, unlike in animals, the relationship between social isolation and addiction is bi-directional in humans. Social isolation leads to addiction and addiction is highly stigmatizing and abhorrent to society. This leads to further social exclusion of these people, which worsens the chances of their breaking free of the grip of addiction, thus creating a vicious cycle.

~

Dr Johl sees a way out of this quagmire. He has formally submitted a blueprint (several times), to the government to pull the state out of the economic mess. It essentially involves taking medium-scale clean industry to villages and establishing 'farm service centres', which the farmer could approach for getting his farm tilled, harvested and the stubble taken out, at charges approved by the government.

'To be able to use technology every farmer does not have to own these machines,' Dr Johl insisted.

'Why does the government not act on the blueprint?' I asked.

'Because the bureaucrats think they know everything?'

'And the politicians?'

'No long-distance vision. They can only see as far as the next election,' he put it simply.

I asked him about the addiction situation in the rural heartland in the old days. He told me that he was nineteen years old at the time of the Partition when he moved from a village in Lyallpur in Pakistan to Indian Punjab with his parents. At that time, opium cultivation was allowed in Punjab although a license was required.

'We did not have any money. It was opium that saved us. We had two small fields, in one, we grew sugar cane and in the other opium. Our *baithak* (sitting room) used to be filled with sacks of opium husk, some of which the farm labourers consumed during harvest weeks, after which they worked tirelessly. The wastage of the husk was thrown away, which the donkeys belonging to the kumhars ate, and they worked non-stop too,' he said with a smile.

On a more serious note, he added, 'It was all legal. There was opium all around us, both in the fields and stacked in jute sacks in the house. None of our family members became addicts. Even farm workers who consumed it during harvest season did not become addicts. And now it is illegal and it costs a bomb. Taking it can mean going to jail and yet there are so many addicts. Doctor Sahib, availability of drugs has nothing to do with addiction. Rajasthan grows a whole lot of opium and we do not grow any. If it was availability, why are we addicts and they are not?' he asked.

Neither Dr Johl nor I knew that the country would face a raging pandemic later in the year in 2020. As the economy went on to crash, the agriculture economy would be the only thing to perform not just as well as before but even better. However, in October 2020, without consulting any stake holders, the central government brought in three parliamentary laws which threw open the purchase of all crops to the mercy of market forces, raising the spectre of the Indian government doing away with the MSP. This would have led to corporatisation of agriculture and an even faster 'de-peasantisation' by pushing the farmers into totally unchartered territory and an unheard-of level of social 'anomie'. During the twelve months of widespread protests that followed, helmed by farmers' bodies, thousands of farmers from North India camped on the roads to Delhi and in Delhi, braving harsh weather conditions. Over 700 farmers are said to have died during the agitation.

After a year of protests, the central government took back the unpopular laws as suddenly as it had instituted them because of the looming election season. Sadly, genuine agricultural reforms to diversify agriculture and increase farming income are still pending.

The War on Drugs is a War Against Our Own Young People

In the beginning of the 20th century, America started to place diplomatic pressure on countries across the world to ban three plant products: opium, cocaine and cannabis as well as their laboratory derivatives. The Americans had realized that prohibiting production within America would do little to solve their country's drug problem because drugs would continue to pour in—not just from across the Mexican border, but from all over the world—to quench the huge appetite for drugs in America.

China had its own opium problem and it collaborated with the US in this push. However, European countries including the UK resisted strongly because they had under their control large, colonized countries like India and many other overseas territories, which held the monopoly on the highly lucrative production and trade of opium. Opium was used as an intoxicant as well as exported to Europe and the USA for the then burgeoning pharmaceutical market. And the taxes and the profits from that sprawling opium empire went to the British and other European governments. Britain and France had waged the Second Opium War against China which they had resoundingly won. In 1860, they extracted as part of an extortionate treaty the opening of eleven more Chinese ports to foreign trade and the right of foreigner traders to travel to regions within China, which had been banned by the Chinese government till then.

After World War II, America emerged as an even more powerful and influential nation than before. Much of that influence was used to ram tough international treaties down the throat of the rest of the world, criminalising not just the production and trade of these drugs but even possession of small quantities by individuals for their own use. Consuming these drugs became a jailable crime overnight in many countries of the world.

Like the rest of the world, India too signed two key UN conventions i.e., UN Single Convention, 1961 and UN Vienna Convention on Psychotropic Substances, 1971. The latter additionally prohibited the use and possession of many psychoactive drugs such as amphetamine-type stimulants, barbiturates, benzodiazepines, psychedelics and even medications used in the treatment of addiction (except on prescription). According to these UN conventions and the country-specific drug laws which emerged from these treaties, there is no such thing as licit recreational drug use now. So, the War on Drugs is not a move to end just addiction. According to Johann Hari, 'It is a war to stop all recreational drug use among all human beings everywhere in the world.'

The Indian law which followed as a consequence of India having signed these international treaties and protocols was the Narcotic Drugs and Psychotropic Substances Act, 1985 or the NDPS Act. It consolidates laws about possession, consumption and sale of drugs. This is one of the harshest drug laws in the world. After it came into being, consumption and possession of the smallest amount of any of these drugs (for personal use) became a criminal offence in India. The NDPS Act is a unique law under which proving possession is enough for a conviction. Unlike in other criminal laws, the intent of carrying a drug is irrelevant here because even personal consumption has been criminalized. Even the length of the sentence does not depend upon intent, it is proportionate to the amount of drug seized from a person and no amount is too small for a person to be allowed to go scot-free.

The NDPS Act, promulgated in 1985 and its several subsequent amendments, aims to do two things. Through various provisions like strict liability, difficult bail conditions and harsh sentences, it aims to deter people from trafficking in drugs. Second, at least on paper, the law provides for medical treatment and de-addiction for individuals identified as drug addicts.

According to a report published in 2018 by the Delhi-based legal think tank, the Vidhi Centre for Legal Policy:

1. Of all the cases registered and persons arrested for trafficking of drugs in the whole country during the year 2013-14, more than 40% were from the state of Punjab while Punjab constitutes just 2% of India's population.

2. 71.4% of the accused brought to the special courts between 2013-15 were between 20-40 years of age of which 40% were between 20-30. Thus, a large proportion of people arrested for possessing drugs were young men.

3. The NDPS Act classifies the quantity of illegal intoxicants seized into small, intermediate and commercial quantities. The length of sentence is proportionate to the quantity seized. Most of those arrested in Punjab were caught with small and intermediate quantities. Even when caught with technically intermediate quantities, the quantity bordered on small in a very large number of cases.

In their study of application of the NDPS Act in Punjab, the Vidhi Centre came up with several conclusions, the most startling of which was that a large portion of the thousands arrested in Punjab were addicts and not drug peddlers or smugglers. Hence the title of the Centre's report, 'Addict to Convict'. The manner of application of the NDPS, according to this report, has defeated and continues to defeat the purpose of the Act in Punjab.

The summer of 2014 was an exceptionally terrifying phase for the young men of Punjab. Campaigning for the general elections for the sixteenth Lok Sabha started in March and was in full swing all over the country soon. The party then ruling Punjab seemed to be lagging according to experts. The popular perception was that the high rates of heroin addiction in Punjab was not just because the government was inefficient in controlling the drug mafia but because some of the politicians in power in the state were hand in glove with them. At campaign rallies, opposition leaders relentlessly pointed out that there was no other explanation for the fact that the smuggling of heroin did not show any sign of abating at all. This became the topic of heated debates on television shows and was prominently featured in newspapers. Snide jokes were made and humorous ditties coined, which then went viral on social media, heaping ridicule on the ruling party members.

The Election Commission of India appointed teams during the campaign for the parliamentary elections to intercept cash and narcotics as these are known to be used by political parties to lure voters. These teams intercepted and seized during the campaign a total of 1.85 lakh kgs of narcotics from the whole country. Out of this, 1.39 lakh kgs were just from Punjab.

The election results were declared on May 14. The opposition party in the state won nine of the thirteen seats in Parliament. Worst for the ruling party was the stinging defeat Arun Jaitley of the BJP suffered in Amritsar. This was the future finance minister of India who enjoyed the support of the then ruling party of Punjab. Whatever may have been the truth, the opposition parties had succeeded in creating a perception that the sitting government was part of the problem, not the solution. Humiliated, the state government responded in a kneejerk manner by ordering large-scale searches and arrests all over the state.

While driving back from my clinic every evening, I would see scooters and motorcycles lined up by the roadside, being searched at the multiple roadblocks which had come up suddenly. Cars were not stopped. Mine never was and I do not even use the 'doctor' sticker on my windscreen. Anybody who tells you drug addiction in Punjab, particularly the law enforcement side of it, is not a class issue, is either ignorant or is lying. It very much is.

Young girls in the cities of Punjab who drive scooters often tie a scarf around their face to protect themselves from the wind, the summer sun and the ever-present dust and smoke polluting the air. It also gives them some degree of anonymity and hence some sense of safety. At the police *nakas* as these roadblocks were called, they were asked to remove their scarves. They also had to open the lid of the storage space in their scooters so the policemen could check them. I never saw any women cops at those roadblocks.

These girls were coming back from work and looked clearly embarrassed emptying their storage space and fishing out half-eaten tiffins, their shopping bags which sometimes included personal items like undergarments, packets of noodles, headache tablets (whose presence had to be explained), menstrual pads, etc., in full view of not just the policemen but the curious passers-by and drivers.

Boys were treated even worse. They were shouted at by impatient policemen and pushed around if there was the slightest delay in producing the registration papers of their vehicles, since the line of scooters to be checked would be getting longer. The red-faced government, determined to show that it was cracking down on smugglers, arrested thousands of young men who were carrying small amounts of heroin, poppy husk, ganja or a few Lomotil tablets. The real dealers and the smugglers were nowhere to be found!

~

Less than a week after the election results were declared, one late afternoon, a nineteen-year-old boy in handcuffs with a fuzzy beard and a shabby turban which had come loose, was pushed into my office by a policeman. The officer of the law was reeking of alcohol and appeared to be chewing tobacco. They were trailed by the boy's father, his face marked by lines of despair and fatigue. The boy had been caught at a barricade that morning with four grams of smack and was being taken to the jail as ordered by the magistrate.

On the way to the jail, they had stopped at a *dhaba* (roadside eatery) for lunch, where, in lieu of half a bottle of liquor, the father had persuaded the officer to stop at my clinic for some medicines, which could help his cold turkey son survive till the bail hearing. I quickly did what I could for the boy's anticipated pains and runny bowels and sent them off with a prescription since the tobacco-chewing officer was clearly in a hurry to go home after dumping the boy in jail.

'With four lousy grams of smack, he could not be peddling,' I said that evening to Bobby, my friend and colleague, who had invited me to his club for a drink. 'Jail? For god's sake! A nineteen-year-old kid! What wrong did he do other than what you, me and that policeman do every other day? And the drunk cop was on duty!'

Bobby spoke slowly and indulgently to me as if addressing a child, 'What that kid did is inexcusable. Addiction has its rules. There is a substance and more importantly, there is style. An etiquette which has to be followed.' *Saleeka* was the actual word he used. 'He makes the rest of us look bad. He is not our kind of addict. That is why society needs to put him away.'

Bobby's sardonic humour reminded me again that only two-wheelers were stopped by the police at the roadblocks and not cars.

Several weeks later, I asked a police officer who had come to my clinic for his wife's treatment about this. He said cars were stopped when there was some specific information, but scooters and motorcycles were stopped as a matter of routine. That is the way it had always been. They did not have enough manpower to check all the vehicles. It would also cause traffic jams; cars occupy a lot of space, the policeman reasoned.

In 2014, 17,084 young men were arrested in Punjab for drug offences which constituted 41% of all such arrests in India. Almost all the arrests were made at roadblocks in cities, towns and the link roads connecting villages. In 2014 alone, the rate of reported NDPS crimes jumped to 50.5 per 100,000 population—four times that of second ranked Maharashtra with a rate of 12.4.

A month after the incident at the clinic, I was in the district court as a medical witness to depose that a patient of mine whose husband had sued for divorce on the grounds of my patient's mental illness was treated by me just for depression and had now completely recovered. While waiting for the case to be heard, I saw the boy who had been brought to my clinic in handcuffs being herded into the court room along with about twenty other young men (all of whom were of roughly the same age). It was a bail hearing, which I came to know later, was postponed because the judge had reported sick.

While the young men were being herded away by the police, I ran into the boy's father. He looked like he had aged several years since we last met and he seemed completely baffled. I had read up about the NDPS Act and had discussed it with my colleagues who had come across similar cases. The law, for all its shortcomings, clearly provided that persons who claimed to be addicted and were caught with small quantities of drugs for their own use were immune from prosecution if they were willing to undergo treatment. The magistrates who tried persons caught with small quantities had the power to refer them for treatment.

I mentioned this to the boy's father along with the fact that his son was caught with four grams of heroin and up to five grams was considered 'small quantity', but I was not sure if the man understood any of it in his anxious state. I advised him to talk to his lawyer and left. I have no idea what happened to that particular boy, but I do know that out of the thousands arrested with small quantities of drugs, not even one person was granted immunity from prosecution and sent for treatment.

The Vidhi Centre report published in April 2018 concluded: 'Based on our data, no person has been sent to de-addiction centres by any court in Punjab under Sections 39 and Section 64A of the NDPS act, which allow addicts to be diverted out of the criminal justice system. These sections have been reduced to dead letters on paper. Addiction continues to be viewed as a criminal offence. The police, prosecution and courts, entrenched in the mindset of the criminal justice system, have failed to treat addiction as a health issue that needs medical care and not criminalization. Various government-appointed committees too have pointed out that addiction is a health problem and not a criminal offence, but this has been ignored.'

Even judges of higher courts are often guided by their moral compass than by scientific evidence or by the law that they are supposed to uphold. Thus, as recently as in May 2019, a two-judge bench of the Punjab & Haryana High Court passed a judgement castigating the police for 'going soft on the addicts' and catching only the smugglers when according to the NDPS Act, consumption of illicit substances is a crime too. It ordered the police officers '...to initiate criminal proceedings against consumers of narcotic drugs and psychotropic substances to eradicate the menace,' totally ignoring the fact that the same NDPS Act also said that addicts were immune from prosecution if they volunteered for treatment. And also that addictions are as much of a medical illness as alcoholism, which is just another name for alcohol addiction. To jail a person for one and to hospitalise a person for the other requires a special kind of split in societal logic.

As mentioned earlier, the NDPS Act is fundamentally different from other laws in the criminal justice system. Here, mere possession of even a miniscule quantity of any of the drugs on the list is a crime, whatever the intention may be. However, as pointed out by Lawyers' Collective, the law does allow for transport and use of narcotic drugs and psychotropic substances for medical and scientific purposes for which licensing and permissions from government agencies are required.

According to the Vidhi Centre report, under other laws, the intention to commit a crime must be proved by the prosecution. Here, however, intention is presumed and hence, does not need to be proved. This is called 'strict liability'. Strict liability provisions do not consider *mens rea* (the intent of causing harm or wrongdoing) and rely solely on *actus reus* (the criminal act) to convict for an offence according to the report. Since intent is harder to prove than a criminal act alone, strict liability provisions ensure higher convictions. The onus of proving absence of criminal intent is on the accused, not on the prosecution. As they lead to a higher rate of conviction, provisions of strict liability are largely viewed as a deterrent.

Rates of conviction under the NDPS Act are much higher as compared to other laws because of this alone. By focusing on possession alone, the Act fails to distinguish between different kinds of crimes (drug consumption, unauthorized possession, peddling, transportation, trafficking, trading, production, etc.) and different kind of offenders (first-time offenders, casual users, drug addicts and trafficking units). Since the law does not require enforcement agencies to establish motive or intent behind said possession, and they still get their convictions, this has led to the police in Punjab adopting a template-based copy paste narrative while filing first information reports (FIRs), across all districts for possession of widely different types and quantities of drugs.

Since the police did not have to prove anything, the quality of investigation nosedived, and they became lazy. Despite the virtual absence of investigation, they still got a high number of convictions, but the sloppy investigation meant that they did not have a clue about the source of drugs or how to nail the real traffickers and smugglers who got away. The jails were filled with young men many of whom were caught carrying drugs for their own or a friend's use. Out of the 13,350 NDPS cases across Punjab studied by the lawyers who wrote the Vidhi report, in 10,959, the FIRs were exactly similar down to every word, comma and full stop—obviously, a copy paste job.

The NDPS Act provides that when a person is caught on suspicion of possessing drugs, it is his right to be searched in the presence of a gazetted officer of a non-police department or a magistrate. It seems that in a touching gesture of abiding trust in the constabulary, who had just waylaid, pursued and caught them, all the 13,350 men waved this statutory right and expressed full faith in the police and allowed to be willingly searched without the presence of a civilian officer, a provision mandated by the law to ensure fair play. The typical template used in these thousands of FIRs was this:

'Police officials were on patrolling duty in connection with checking of bad character persons. One gentleman was seen approaching, carrying in his right hand, a glazed paper bag. On seeing the police party, he tried to turn right under suspicious circumstances. The Assistant Sub-Inspector, based on suspicion, intercepted him with the help of other team members. The accused was asked to clarify his 'whereabouts'(?). Then, the officer informed the accused of his suspicion regarding some intoxicant substance that was inside the glazed paper carry bag. The accused was further informed that he had a legal right to be searched in the presence of a gazetted officer or magistrate. The accused reposed confidence in the police officer. On search, intoxicating powder was found in the plastic envelope which was seized.'

Interestingly, in 100% of cases, which numbered tens of thousands, all the accused were carrying the plastic envelope in their right hand or in their right pocket while about 20% of any population, (males even more than females), is left-handed!

Inevitably, jails in Punjab became overcrowded and continue to be so. According to data gathered in 2015, against a total capacity of 18,629, the jails in Punjab had 23,421 prisoners out of which roughly 40% were in jail for drug-related offences while the remaining 60% were jailed for all other offences combined. 41% of those who were imprisoned for drug offences were undertrials awaiting trial because of the harsh bail provisions.

According to the report released by the National Crime Records Bureau (NCRB) in 2017, Maharashtra reported the highest number of FIRs under the Narcotics Drugs and Psychotropic Substances Act (NDPS) with 14,634 cases, followed by Punjab (12,356 cases) in the second place. The NCRB data states that 5,913 out of 12,356 FIRs were lodged for possession of drugs for the purpose of trafficking in Punjab. The remaining 6,443 FIRs filed in Punjab pertained to possessing small amounts of drugs for personal consumption. For Maharashtra, as many as 14,097 cases out of 14,634 (a whopping 96.33%), were lodged for possessing small amounts of drugs for personal use.

However, the fact remains that since 2002, despite high convictions owing to strict liability provisions and despite harsh bail rules, jails continue to be packed with persons accused of drug offences—contributing almost as many inmates as those accused of all other offences combined. It appears that the Act has failed to act as deterrent on the ground. One of the reasons is that the 'presumed guilt' provisions assuring convictions resulting in shoddy template-based investigation, the origins of drugs become a secondary aim and thus paradoxically, the real purpose of the NDPS Act is defeated.

According to the NCRB, 59,806 cases were registered under the NDPS Act in the whole of the country in 2020, out of which 33,246 were for possession of drugs for personal use and for consumption and a lesser number—26,560—for possession of drugs for trafficking. Nothing is a more telling indicator of the stark reality of the justice system being focused more on the users than the traffickers. Punjab continued to be in second place in 2020, next to UP, which has a population about seven times that of Punjab. As many as 4,039 cases were registered under the NDPS in Punjab.

The ratio of smugglers/sellers to consumers arrested continues to be dismal for most of India. Numbers also tell us how unsuccessful the Mumbai police has been. Arrests for personal consumption accounted for 93.3% of all arrests in Mumbai under the NDPS Act in 2020. According to Neha Singhal of the Vidhi Centre for Legal Policy, 99% of all arrests under the NDPS Act in Mumbai are of marginalized people (labourers, rickshaw drivers and delivery boys). Carrying this to an absurd level, the Hyderabad police on October 28, 2021 began to stop youngsters on the road and check their phones for messages to see if they had tried to procure ganja, thus making a mockery of not just the Supreme Court mandated right to privacy but also of the common law of the country by trying to make WhatsApp messages proof of consumption.

The idea is not necessarily to justify what youngsters do but that the real issue of drugs and of those involved in the business, its transportation and distribution of fatal drugs such as heroin gets lost. The purpose seems to be just to arrest a large number of people under the NDPS Act as a showpiece for television news and for political purposes. Television channels lap this up since it increases their ratings by assuaging the morality of the average viewer.

The drugs issue has been so heavily politicized that every now and then the politicians in power in states as well as at the centre make regular claims trying to outdo one another in a bidding war of sorts, citing the numbers of people arrested by them to wipe out the scourge of drugs. All these numbers are in tens of thousands and a vast majority of them are users and not smugglers.

~

India copied America's War on Drugs at a huge cost to the country both in terms of money and human misery. This money should have been spent on rehabilitation and treatment of drug addicts and on alleviating the pain of the families of persons with addiction. Ironically, while we continue to be firmly entrenched in this war against persons with drug addiction, America is reconsidering its position, and the realization that war is something that is waged against other countries and not against its own people, is sinking in.

In 2011, the Global Commission on Drug Policy released a critical report on the War on Drugs, declaring: 'The global War on Drugs has failed, with devastating consequences for individuals and societies around the world. Sixty years after the UN Single Convention on Narcotic Drugs and fifty years after President Nixon launched the US government's War on Drugs, fundamental reforms in national and global drug control policies are urgently needed.'

Former US President Jimmy Carter wrote an op-ed in *The New York Times* strongly endorsing the recommendations of the commission, saying they were in line with the policies of his administration. Carter went on to say it was the policies of the succeeding Reagan administration which had moved US policy so far toward punitive alternatives. The US seems to have realized that the country committed and perpetuated a huge blunder for more than a hundred years at a massive financial and human cost. Early signs of a sensible US retreat from that 'War' are there for all to see.

Twenty-one states and the District of Columbia in the United States have legalized recreational use of marijuana. So have countries like Canada, Georgia, South Africa, Uruguay, Spain, Belize, the Czech Republic, Costa Rica, Columbia and the Australian Capital Territory in Australia. Switzerland, the Netherlands and Portugal too have decriminalized personal use and possession of small amounts of drugs.

It is hard not to point out the similarity between how

Indian society treats persons with addiction with how it treated persons with homosexual orientation till very recently. Britain, a colonial western power, made homosexuality a crime in India in 1861, based on Christian religious beliefs. And it was made a jailable offence by instituting Section 377 in the Indian Penal Code. In 1947, the British left India. Even after independence, India continued with Section 377. In 1967, the British decriminalized gay sex in their own country but India persisted with it for another fifty years before the courts struck it off the statute book in 2018.

In the same manner, the harsh drug laws imposed by the West continue in India without any hope of moderation while the West has revised its opinion. The West has not just started thinking on more progressive and scientific lines but has actually liberalized drug use to a significant extent and continues to bring in more liberalising measures. On the contrary, India is instituting measures even harsher than the notoriously harsh NDPS.

In December 2018, the Punjab government announced the setting up of an Advisory Board to enable detention of drug peddlers and smugglers for a year without trial. If past history is any indication, a majority of them will again be young men who are users and small-time peddlers carrying drugs for themselves and sometimes also for their peer addicts.

Maybe it is time to realise that if ratcheting up the harshness of legal measures has not worked in reducing the social and individual pathology called addiction, a fresh approach is required. In addition to the supply side, it is time to focus on the demand side. It is crucial to recognise that even a small liberal step goes a long way in lessening social stigma attached to addictions, which are essentially chronic diseases with a remitting and relapsing course, needing treatment, not prison sentences.

CHAPTER 5

Why are Cannabis and Opium 'Drugs' and Alcohol and Tobacco Not?

In Chapter 4, I mentioned how a nineteen-year-old boy along with his anxious father was herded into my clinic by a policeman, who was drunk and also chewing tobacco. The arrested boy was being taken to jail for carrying four grams of smack, just about enough for four days' use. The police had confiscated it when the boy was caught at a barricade on the street and he was in withdrawal. What stayed with me was the irony of the situation. A law enforcement officer under the effect of two drugs—tobacco and alcohol—was taking to jail a young man for having used and carried a third drug; while medical experts around the world would agree that the drugs used by that policeman are far more harmful than the one used by the young boy.

Cannabis, cocaine, opium, morphine, tobacco, alcohol, caffeine are all drugs, as are heroin, methamphetamine and many others. All of these act on the brain and alter consciousness. None are harmful if taken once in a while. All can be abused and lead to addiction. All are sources of profit.

However, the so-called War on Drugs, unleashed by the US-sponsored United Nations treaties between 1961 and 1988, has been strangely selective. It has created a world in which tobacco and liquor are legally available for consumption at street corners while consumption of ganja, opium or cocaine or carrying these for one's own use is a crime punishable with jail sentence.

Is there even a shred of scientific or medical logic behind this arrangement? The answer is 'absolutely none'!

In his book, *Forces of Habit*, David T. Courtwright says that alcohol, tobacco and caffeine were the 'big three' drugs even before the worldwide prohibition in 1961 of the 'little three' i.e. opium, cannabis and cocaine. The sheer scale of production, distribution and consumption of the 'big three' and the degree to which they were integrated into cultures around the world made them immune to being banned. Alcohol and cigarettes had been normalized and were part of the romantic and sexual landscape of the then modern society. Tweeds smelling of tobacco were fetishized, 'cigarette breath' a romantic given and the 'one after', a normative sexual ritual. Alcohol was a sexual facilitator and sexist vodka advertisements carrying the caption, 'liquid panty remover' could be seen in chic magazines. An urban subculture had sprung up with norms like wine with meals, coffee after meals and beer with darts and pool as its markers. It would have been not just global commercial suicide for regimes across the world to prohibit alcohol and tobacco when they prohibited the 'little three' but also cultural suicide for the 'brave new world' of that time.

Cultural linkages with local drugs existed in the non-western world as well. Bhang, ganja and charas have been part of religious rituals and festivities in India for centuries and cannabis is associated with Lord Shiva in the public consciousness. Consumption of bhang during Holi in North India is a well-accepted part of the festival and many Bollywood

Holi songs contain reference to it. Opium has been used ritually in Rajasthan during festivals, family ceremonies and as an offering to guests.

It is often said that when you cannot find the logic behind something, follow the money. Many think that cannabis and opium were banned because the international alcohol and tobacco lobby feared competition in the not-too-distant future from these two drugs. Opium, cannabis and coca—the 'little three'—were far less frequently consumed than alcohol, tobacco and caffeine and 'reformers' eventually succeeded in making them illegal. Since these are illegal and prohibited, most people think of these when they hear the word 'drugs.'

In 1961, at the time of the Single Convention to prohibit drugs, America knew from its own experience from 1920-33 that prohibition of alcohol was catastrophic to law and order and the economics of a society. It was also no secret that it makes societies poorer and lawless without necessarily turning them healthier or more moral.

Did the western world know then that criminalising opium, cannabis and cocaine may backfire like prohibition of alcohol did in the USA a few years back? Those who ran the world at that time—diplomats, businessmen and politicians—were wise and balance people. So, they certainly would have known although they may not have anticipated the degree to which banning these three and waging a war against them would eventually harm societies around the world.

However, while people everywhere needed their intoxicants, reformists had to be mollified and business choices were to be made. Something had to be sacrificed on the global altar of morality. Post-World War II, the USA had emerged as a very powerful country and the newly constituted UN, funded mainly by the USA, needed to take up work for global good.

However, a serious concern has been nagging students of drug history since then. In the history of civilizations, whenever a drug proved to be a nuisance either for people's physical or mental health, for law and order or for morality, the establishment taxed it even more, not banned it. That took care of demand and nobody would be poorer. This was a far more sophisticated strategy, which was commercially sound and equally effective.

Why was the same strategy not used then? Was it because taxing opium, cocaine and cannabis would not have satisfied the reformers or soothed moral outrage? Far more cogent is the argument that most of the distilling and brewing happened in the West and most of the tobacco corporations too were based there while none of the decision-making western countries grew the three drugs (opium, cannabis and coca) listed on the 'to be banned' list. They were all products of the eastern, not the western world. The countries which grew these had been colonies of the West but were no longer so, and any tax imposed now would not go to the former colonisers in the West.

Thus, in an irony of history, Britain became an international controller of opium from being the biggest trafficker of the drug in human history. Overnight, the trafficker, which had used its military and navy to wage two big wars against China so that it could sell massive amounts of opium in China (while opium was illegal there) to shore up its own sagging economy, turned into an anti-opium crusader and enforcer.

~

Most popular narratives, commentaries, documentaries and movies with drugs as the theme mention neither alcohol nor tobacco as a drug, implicitly or explicitly. When the popular war cry, 'Say No to Drugs' is sounded from any podium, alcohol and tobacco are far from the speakers' or listeners' minds. Most people do not expect to find alcohol on any list of drugs. Because drugs are something that 'others do in dark alleys and ramshackle buildings'.

One of the reasons for this utterly naïve perception is that alcohol is a liquid which comes with fancy packaging. The fact, however, is that alcohol is a drug, the full chemical name of which is ethyl alcohol and if it came in the form of capsules or injections, there would probably have been less difficulty in perceiving it as a drug. People wonder: how could alcohol be a drug when it is legal, comes in elegant bottles and sold openly at duty-free arcades and shopping malls? How could something sharing the menu along with tea and lemonade in five-star restaurants be a drug? The state law is at work here in changing public opinion as a social engineer. If in addition to being available as capsules or injections, alcohol was illegal and consuming or selling it invited arrest and imprisonment for ten years under the NDPS Act, nobody would have a problem calling alcohol a drug.

According to various estimates, at least 2,000 million people throughout the world regularly use alcohol and just about 13.5 million people use opioids. Global alcohol consumption has increased in recent decades, with most or all of this increase occurring in developing countries. According to a 2002 WHO report, alcohol caused 1.8 million deaths in a year worldwide and was estimated to cause, worldwide, 20–30% of oesophageal cancer, liver disease, epilepsy, motor vehicle accidents and homicide and other intentional injuries.

National Drug Survey, 2019 found that alcohol was the most commonly used as well as the most commonly abused 'drug' in India. Sixteen crore Indians used alcohol as compared to 3.1 crore who used cannabis and 2.2 crore who used opioids, making alcohol by far the highest used intoxicant in the country. Punjab ranked third among all Indian states after Chhattisgarh and Tripura with 28.5% people who used alcohol against the national prevalence of 14.6%. Punjab's prevalence of drinking was a half percent more than that of much-maligned Goa. More than half the males in Punjab drank socially.

About half of the people who drank either had medical problems because of drinking or had history of physical fights, daytime drinking or traffic accidents under the influence. Punjab also has the dubious distinction of having the highest prevalence of drinking by minors at 6%, which is more than four times the national average of 1.3%. The rest of the country, through the lens of popular media, sees Punjab as a drug-ravaged state not because so many adults and minors drink, but because so many people use heroin. Subtract heroin from the equation and Punjab will have as shiny an image as it had forty years back.

On the other hand, in the context of drugs, nobody has even heard the name of the Indian state of Chhattisgarh, which not only has the highest proportion of population which drinks but also the second highest proportion of women who drink. Why is this so? Because alcohol is not considered a drug!

~

Several studies published in the late 1990s reported that red wine in moderation might be good for your heart. Hardly any other medical study has been received with more cheer across the world. The mainstream media featured it prominently and it is safe to assume that the wine producers of the world did their part in spreading the good word too. Somewhere down the line, it came down to the notion that it was alcohol which was beneficial when taken in moderate amounts whether it was wine or beer or spirits. Again, there were sane voices cautioning that it could be just the marketing genius of beer, whiskey and vodka manufacturing companies at work. But the belief that two drinks a day was better for your health than not drinking at all stuck. Many men displayed newspaper cuttings on their refrigerators at home to convince their wives they drank for health reasons and not for fun.

However, the bad news for those who enjoy a drink or two is this: *The Lancet* carried another study in 2018 and concluding its extensive report, the authors wrote, 'The safest level of drinking is none.' Dr Atul Ambekar of the All India Institute of Medical Sciences (AIIMS), New Delhi further contextualized this study:

'Research has established that the risk of health damage increases manifold with higher levels of consumption of alcohol. However, in the Indian context, the level of alcohol consumption above which there is a high risk of health damage is not yet determined. So, it is difficult to suggest a safe level of consumption anywhere but more so in India.

However, if one still wants to drink, the latest medical advice is for men to stick to six to seven drinks per week, which is one drink a day. It is less harmful but still there is a risk. For women, the recommendation is three to four drinks per week, because they metabolize alcohol slower as compared to men and so it stays that much longer in the body.'

Trying to convince Indians that one drink means 35 ml and not 60 or 70 ml, as they have always believed it to be, is a Herculean job. In the case of beer, it is a 330 ml bottle which constitutes one drink and not the bigger 660 ml one. For wine, it is 150 ml.

Most people in India are not enamoured by such small quantities. As one of my patients said testily, 'It is easier not to drink than to drink so little.' There is also the fact to consider that Indians drink alcohol very differently from the rest of the world. According to the National Drug Survey 2019, even among those Indians who drink occasionally or 'socially', about half of them, whenever they do drink, consume more than four drinks in one sitting, a pattern called Heavy Episodic Drinking. Almost as a sacrosanct cultural norm, an Indian would drink before—rather than along with or after meals, which makes the rate of absorption much faster than the human body can metabolise (which is just one drink of 35 ml of whiskey per hour).

In another study funded by the Bill and Melinda Gates Foundation published in *The Lancet* in July 2022, the authors studied data from across the world and reported that the population-level health risks associated with low levels of alcohol consumption were far greater for younger populations than for older ones. Emmanuela Gakidou, Professor of Health Metrics Sciences and Senior Director of Organizational Development and Training at the Institute for Health Metrics and Evaluation (IHME), University of Washington, says, 'While it may not be realistic to think young adults will abstain from drinking, it is important to communicate the latest evidence so that everyone can make informed decisions about their health.'

There is not a vital organ of the body from the liver to the nerves to the brain to the digestive system and hormones, which alcohol does not damage in the long run. Alcohol significantly increases the chances of many cancers in addition to being by far the most common cause of fatal liver damage. Alcohol is the only drug which in addition to being harmful to the individual can directly cause death and disability to others via traffic accidents.

~

David Nutt is Professor of Neuropsychopharmacology at Imperial College London. Before 2007, he was also Chairman of the UK Government's Advisory Council on the Misuse of Drugs (ACMD), in short, the UK government's advisor-in-chief on drugs. During his stint as advisor to the UK government, he conducted a significant study. After going through all available research on every recreational drug and calculating how likely it was to harm you and to cause you to harm other people, he allotted a composite score to each drug, indicating degree of self-harm plus harm to others. Professor Nutt found that one drug was far ahead of others with a harm score of 72. The second-most harmful drug (to self and others) was heroin with a harm score of 55 just ahead of crack cocaine with a score of 54 and methamphetamine at 32. The most harmful drug with the score 72 was alcohol. Professor Nutt clarified that it was not that other drugs were safe—they certainly were not, but alcohol was even more dangerous.

Two important events occurred after the publication of this report in 2007. Professor Nutt was fired by the UK government from the post of advisor-in-chief on drugs. In a letter the home secretary expressed 'surprise and disappointment over Professor Nutt's report, which damaged efforts to give the public clear messages about the dangers of drugs. We remain determined to crack down on all *illegal* substances and minimise their harm to health and society.' Please note the emphasis on the words 'illegal substances'. A news report in *The Guardian* was headlined 'Professor David Nutt Asked to Resign after his Claims that Ecstasy and LSD were Less Dangerous than Alcohol.'

The second important event related to Professor Nutt's report and his subsequent dismissal by the UK government was that he received the prestigious international award, the John Maddox Prize for Standing up for Science. The judges awarded the Prize to Professor Nutt 'in recognition of the impact his thinking and actions have had in influencing evidence-based classification of drugs in the United Kingdom and elsewhere in the world, and his continued courage and commitment to rational debate, despite opposition and public criticism.'

In Professor Nutt's list of four drugs most harmful to self and others there is a drug missing, which was not included in the study. If included, it would have received a score much higher than even alcohol. That drug is tobacco. Tobacco is a legal drug like alcohol but unlike alcohol, it cannot be consumed in public places now in many countries (at least by smoking), and has been carrying health warnings for decades on its packets long before alcohol bottles did because of the health hazards posed to self, and to others from passive smoking. It is now well known that tobacco is not just the cause of a disproportionately large number of cases of cancers, but also of disability and deaths because of heart and chest diseases.

A later study led by Professor Nutt following a similar methodology and published in *The Lancet* in November 2010 reiterated that alcohol was the most harmful drug in Britain, scoring 72 out of a possible 100, which made it far more damaging than heroin (55) or crack cocaine (54) if both harm to self and to others in society are calculated. It is the most harmful to others by a wide margin, and for harm to the individual alone, it is ranked fourth, behind heroin, crack and methamphetamine (crystal meth).

Ironically, tobacco and alcohol, the two most harmful drugs to human beings as assessed by medical evidence are legal, while the much less harmful drugs are illegal. This is not an argument for prohibition of alcohol because there is impeccable historical evidence that what prohibition of alcohol does is much worse than what alcohol does, both to the individual and the society.

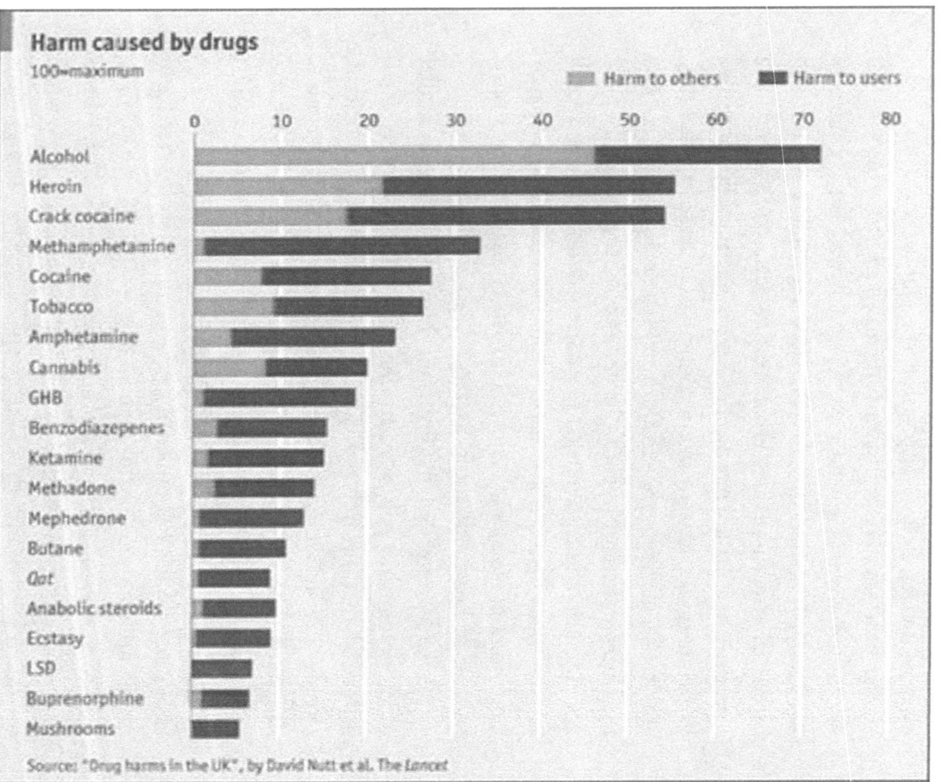
Harm caused by drugs
100=maximum
Harm to others
Harm to users
0
10
20
30
40
50
60
70
80
Alcohol
Heroin
Crack cocaine
Methamphetamine
Cocaine
Tobacco
Amphetamine
Cannabis
GHB
Benzodiazepenes
Ketamine
Methadone
Mephedrone
Butane
Qat
Anabolic steroids
Ecstasy
LSD
Buprenorphine
Mushrooms
Source: "Drug harms in the UK", by David Nutt et al. The Lancet

All that prohibition of any drug does is push it underground and bootlegging makes the drug more powerful and the quality dangerous. Thousands are jailed and because of the mafia, the crime rate soars.

The Indian state of Bihar ordered prohibition of alcohol in 2016 and by 2019, 1.67 lakh persons had been arrested for selling or possessing alcohol in their homes. Courts in Bihar are clogged with two lakh prohibition-related cases in addition to 40,000 bail cases related to prohibition pending with high court alone. During a hearing in 2019, the Patna High Court sought a reply from the chief secretary on the pile of prohibition cases before the high court. The court observed that the rate of pendency had become a huge burden for the judiciary in the absence of an adequate number of courts, judges and court staff. In the last five years, 200 people have died after consuming illegally produced hooch since the liquor ban was instituted in 2016.

The National Family Health Survey conducted by the Ministry of Health and Welfare (2019-2021) too found that in all four states—Bihar, Gujarat, Mizoram and Nagaland, which have instituted prohibition, it is creating more problems than solving them.

This is an invitation to consider that what we are witnessing today in India, and particularly in Punjab, in the context of opioids is not because of opioids alone but a combination of the ill effects of opioids and the elaborate, costly and a less than humane system to enforce prohibition of opioids and cannabis, which criminalises consumption of even small amounts.

It is a commonly held notion that heroin is so addictive that if you force a person to use it for three days, he will be asking for it on the fourth. Hence, it is the most addictive drug known, as the argument goes. According to a US national survey, the highest chances of addiction after casual use of any drug is for tobacco. 32% of people who used it even once went on to long-term habitual use. For alcohol, marijuana and cocaine, the rates are almost the same at 15% and for heroin, it is 23%.

The National Survey of India carried out in 2019 records that while 14.6% of people in India used alcohol, 5.2% were problem users. The corresponding figures for cannabis are 2.83 and 0.66 and for opiates, 2.06 and 0.70. Tobacco was not included in this survey but the Global Adult Tobacco Survey India Factsheet of 2016-17 tells us that in India 8.6% of adults (men-15.2%, women-1.7%) smoke tobacco daily while 18.2% of adults use smokeless tobacco (men-25.1%, women-11.1%). It seems while a large number of Indian women are dependent on tobacco, due to stigma, social role expectations and probably workplace restrictions, they prefer to take it by chewing or keeping it in their mouth.

People who work in the field of addiction will tell you that treatment of addictions is frustrating and requires infinite patience on the part of the treating team. They will also tell you that tobacco addiction is one of the most difficult to treat. Anybody who is trying to give up smoking will agree.

There are three important takeaways from these figures:

1. Alcohol and tobacco (not heroin, cocaine or cannabis) are the two most addictive as well as the most medically harmful intoxicants. Both are not just legal but socially sanctioned, encouraged, romanticized and in the case of alcohol, promoted worldwide at the cost of billions of dollars by direct and proxy advertising.

2. These figures tell us that while many people use drugs, the vast majority use them responsibly without being drawn into addiction and problem use. Alcohol and tobacco are freely available, even so the vast majority does not drink or smoke.

3. If such large numbers of people can use drugs and still not get addicted this means that drugs themselves cannot be the sole reason why people get hooked to them. There have to be other more important factors which determine why a minority of users get addicted and the majority does not.

It is important to remember that the single most powerful factor which works against addiction even in the presence of easy availability of a drug is an individual's connectedness to the people around him from the crib to the deathbed.

None of the points made in this chapter should be interpreted to mean that the colossal danger of currently illegal drugs is being discounted by villainising alcohol or tobacco. *All drugs are dangerous.* The only argument being made here is that banning certain drugs and leaving out others by global policy makers has not worked in the last six decades possibly because the selection was not only biased but based on considerations other than scientific. And blanket prohibitions backed by a harsh criminal justice system cannot be the solution. At least, not the *only* solution.

If we compare the usage of the three most common categories of drugs in the 2019 Magnitude survey with another 2004 survey conducted by UNODC and the Ministry of Social Justice and Empowerment, use of alcohol which is legal, seems to have remained stable over the last fifteen years. On the other hand, in spite of the mere use of cannabis and opioids like heroin being a jailable offence, cannabis use has increased by roughly one-and-a-half times, while use of opioid drugs has increased three to four times.

Whether we like it or not, most human beings are going to feel the need for some intoxicants. The only metric in making some of them more available than others should be the degree of harm caused by each intoxicant.

Chapter 6

Politicians' Fanciful Figures and the Real Data

Punjab and Punjabis have always had a larger-than-life image in the national consciousness, which is disproportionate to its size. The state's land area is only 1.53% of the whole country and its population, just 2% of the national population. As they say, Punjab's footprint is bigger than its foot. There are various reasons for this. Pre-Partition Punjab was several times larger than present-day Punjab and anyone whose ancestors hail from there are Punjabis no matter where they live now. A disproportionately large number of Punjabis live outside Punjab. Historically, Punjabis have lived for centuries in a land, which was the gateway to India and was ravaged every time invaders attacked the country. Things had to be rebuilt from scratch every time and there were new people from foreign lands to deal with since many of the invaders stayed back. The people of Punjab have evolved over the centuries to a hardy race fit to fight as well as to assimilate strangers (even the invaders), and learn new skills from them as well as teach them new skills in return.

Sikhs, with their distinct identity and the generous free food for all *langar* culture are often the first responders in times of a crisis. You will see them rushing in to help when any part of India is affected by flood, famine or epidemic. Indian film songs rely on the fast Punjabi beat far more than on any other regional music. Movies with a colourful Punjabi wedding scene are always marketable. Punjab also has a centuries-old intellectual tradition of tolerance, Sufi philosophy and Sufi literature. It is also the breadbasket of India. Even in the current lean times, it contributes 38% of wheat to the national pool, produces 25% of rice and 12% of cereal cultivated in India. This is no mean feat for such a small state. Due to these reasons, whatever happens in Punjab is always in the national spotlight.

When drug addiction in Punjab started peaking at the beginning of the millennium, it attracted attention and was commented upon extensively. Unfortunately, but inevitably, politicians of all hues from the state as well as outside it started talking about dire scenarios, so that they could blame other politicians more effectively. The need for methodical assessments of the extent of the problem, the essential pre-requisite for a systematic solution for any major social issue, was pushed away from public discourse due to this.

In October 2012, Rahul Gandhi, the then General Secretary of the Congress party, visited Chandigarh. In a speech at Punjab University, he made the startling claim that seven out of every ten youths of Punjab were suffering from drug addiction. He did not explain it, nor did he divulge the source from where he had derived this outrageous estimate. Nevertheless, the figure of 70% of Punjab's youth being addicted to drugs stuck around and was quoted far and wide in the following weeks and months. Rahul Gandhi's attack was meant to denigrate the then ruling party of Punjab, the Akali-BJP combine. At the time, one of their ministers, Bikram Singh Majithia, had been accused by the media of being hand in glove with drug dealers.

So, where did Rahul Gandhi get his 70% figure? Did he pluck it out of thin air? Yes and no. A few years prior to his speech, Guru Nanak Dev University, Amritsar had conducted a study of persons with drug addiction and in their sample of 600 addicted persons, 73.5% were between 16-35 years of age. It was not a survey of the general population but just a study of people known to be suffering from addiction. Interestingly, some Punjab government officials took a look at the study at that time, misinterpreted it to mean that more than 70% of youth were addicted to drugs (instead of the fact that more than 70% of those addicted were young people). Panicked officials included the issue of drug addiction in the state government's Disaster Management Plan wherein government files now acknowledged that 'some 73.5% of the state's youth between 16-35 years are confirmed drug addicts.' The state Disaster Management Plan went ahead and categorized drug addiction as a 'hazardous category' of disaster!

Ironically, the Department of Disaster Management was under Majitha, the very minister who was accused, wrongly or rightly, of being in cahoots with the drug mafia. Rahul Gandhi was just quoting a figure from a document generated by the minister's own department, which happened to be wildly off the mark. This incident represents like nothing else could, the bungled approach to the issue and the scant trouble governments take to prepare, obtain or verify data. All sorts of numbers and percentages continue to be bandied around by politicians, government departments and even NGOs working in the field.

Politicians have been belting out various figures about the extent of drug addiction in Punjab and the estimates have varied from negligible to calamitous, depending upon how close the elections are and which political party the leader belongs to.

The pity is that neither the politicians nor the bureaucrats pause to make sense of the data they are brandishing. Experts are clear that exaggeration of addiction data is counter-productive because it stigmatises the whole society and leads to pessimism and policy paralysis.

Even when reliable data about the incidence of drug addiction was available, this did not find its rightful place in the state government's files to drive policy making, either about demand reduction or supply reduction of drugs. Supply reduction is about reducing the illegal supply of drugs resulting in reduced availability, while demand reduction is about people looking less for drugs as a result of awareness or the persons with addiction receiving effective treatment and not needing drugs any longer. Supply reduction is usually under the police department and demand reduction, under the department of health.

Before any country, state or community can even start planning an initiative to tackle a problem, in this case, addiction, it is crucial to first narrow down the narrative to the exact extent of the problem. This is to ensure that the planners are neither paralysed by doomsday prophecies nor reassured by the 'everything is fine, we will solve it in six months' type of promises.

One good way of doing it is to focus on a population survey conducted jointly by the Ministry of Social Justice and Empowerment, Government of India and the National Drug Dependence Treatment Centre, AIIMS, New Delhi in February 2019. The study report is titled 'Magnitude of Substance Use in India'. (I have referred to it simply as the National Survey or Magnitude Survey at some places in this book). This was the first time in the history of the country an effort was made to study and document substance use in all the states and union territories at one go. The project remains the only comprehensively done countrywide simultaneous survey of all drugs, including alcohol (but excluding tobacco), led jointly by a team of academicians/clinicians at AIIMS and the Social Justice Ministry.

From conception to conclusion the project took three years. And it was conducted simultaneously in all thirty-six states and union territories of India. More than 1,500 mental health workers were involved in the countrywide data collection exercise, which was done between December 2017 and October 2018. The surveyors visited more than two lakh households and interviewed a total of 473,569 individuals between 10-75 years of age. They asked the respondents about eight categories of drugs: alcohol, cannabis, opioids, cocaine, amphetamine type stimulants, sedatives, inhalants and hallucinogens. While the survey included alcohol, it excluded nicotine.

A large majority of Indians were found to have been drug-naïve in the sense that they had never used any of these eight drugs. The ones who had exposure to drugs were divided into the following categories:

1. *Current User* was somebody who had used it at least once in the last one year. The word 'user' is synonymous with 'current'. It can be argued that if someone had a beer six months back or a glass of bhang on the previous Holi ten months back, and nothing since then, he could hardly be given the label of 'current user' of alcohol or bhang. However, this is not about individuals. When the report says that 14.6% of Indians had one drink or more in the last one year, what it is also eloquently saying is that for all practical purposes, almost as many as 85.4% of the people in India are teetotallers.

2. *Harmful Use* is current use of a drug, along with scores higher than a given cut off on a screening test, which rates:
    i) a person's health

ii) and if there have been interpersonal, social, legal or financial problems related to drug use in the last three months.

3. *Dependence* is defined as current use of the substance along with higher scores on a screening test for dependence and implies the person finds it unable to carry on without regularly using the drug.

According to the survey, 'for most substances, a minority of users met the threshold for harmful use and dependence'. However, the proportion of harmful or dependent users varied between different substances, indicating the different propensity of various substances to lead to dependence and/or health/social problems. The sum of estimates of harmful and dependent use represents the 'quantum of work' for the health and social welfare sectors implying proportion of population which needs help.

Both the categories of dependence and of harmful use need treatment and in an ideal world, should receive treatment when they ask for it. These two categories together are sometimes called 'problem use' implying that the drug use is problematic and is beyond being just recreational. Knowing the numbers of problem users is important because these are the numbers which should drive the policy decisions of governments rather than bursts of moral panic, real or contrived, triggered by politicians from time to time.

Let us look at the numbers countrywide and see how various Indian states compare regarding the numbers of problem users of various drugs. Although the study surveyed both sexes between the age of 10-75 years, a striking but not very surprising finding was that drug use in India is mainly a phenomenon that affects adult men.

Alcohol

According to the survey, 14.6% of all Indians between the ages of 10-75 years had used alcohol in the previous one year, out of which most were males. 27.3% of all males and just 1.6% of all females in the country had consumed alcohol at least once in the previous one year.

One out of five male users suffer from alcohol dependence, while only one in sixteen alcohol-using women are dependent on it.

Looking at it from the opposite perspective, three-fourth of all Indian males and 98.4% of all Indian females had not touched alcohol in the previous one year.

Breaking it up age-wise, 1.3% of all minors (below 18 years) in the country have used alcohol in the last one year. People who use alcohol appear to be evenly distributed across socio-economic classes. *Drinking or not drinking is not a class issue. Both rich and poor drink equally. It is just the type of beverage which is different.*

Country liquor or *desi sharaab* and Indian Made Foreign Liquor, an oxymoronic term firmly entrenched in the Indian excise system as IMFL, were the two most preferred alcoholic beverages among current users at about 30% each. 11% drank homemade alcoholic beverages.

Liquor made in India is classified as beer, country liquor and IMFL. Country liquor is made from a variety of raw materials and has different names in different parts of the country. IMFL is a term used for western-style hard liquors such as whiskey, rum and vodka, which are manufactured in India but do not have any Indian heritage. The term IMFL is used to differentiate these from indigenous recipes such as fenny, toddy and arrack, which are collectively called country liquor.

In a significant finding, fewer Indians drank alcoholic beverages with low alcohol content like beer or wine. The majority of Indians who drink beer prefer strong beer to light beer and only 4% of those who drink, drink wine. In the Northeastern states, there was a strong preference for homemade rice beer. However, the highest proportion of people drinking illicit distilled liquor (*kuccha sharaab, hooch*) was reported from the state of Bihar which has been under prohibition since 2016. This is an example of how banning an intoxicant makes it stronger and more dangerous. While a majority of those who drink also use tobacco, very few (6.4%) of them reported using illegal drugs.

How do these figures compare internationally? According to a 2018 WHO report, 'current use' of alcohol in persons above fifteen years is more than 50% globally as compared to only 14.6% of Indians. But when it comes to harmful use and problem drinking, prevalence of problem drinking in India (5.2%) is slightly higher than in the rest of the world (5.1%). A fair proportion of alcohol users experience indicators of problematic consumption like 'getting involved in physical fights' after drinking (26.8%), 'daytime consumption of alcohol' (21.2%) and 'road traffic accidents' under the influence of alcohol (4.1%).

Thus, while a much higher proportion of Indians may be teetotallers as compared to the rest of the world, when it comes to harmful and problem drinking Indian figures are slightly worse than the global average. In other words, proportionately fewer Indians drink but more get drunk.

In India, very few people drink beer and of those who do, prefer the extra strong variety and the typical Indian prefers spirits than either beer or wines. Even more telling than the beverages consumed in India, it is the amount consumed by

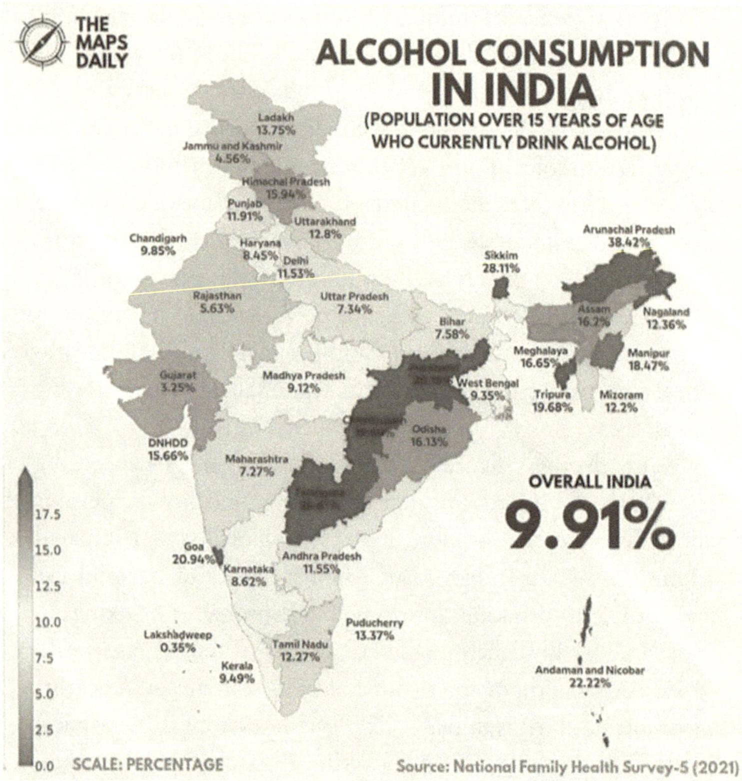

Indians at one sitting. Around half (43%) of alcohol users in India, consume 'more than four drinks on a single occasion'. This pattern of drinking has been named 'Heavy Episodic Drinking' in the survey. It appears that a whole lot of Indians do not touch alcohol at all but a large number among those who drink, drink as if there is no tomorrow. Indians tend to cluster more at the extremes than in the middle when it comes to drinking. India has disproportionately more teetotallers as well as problematic drinkers than the rest of the world. Less Indians proportionately are moderate or sensible drinkers.

This was also the conclusion of the National Family Health Survey conducted by the Union ministry of Health and Family Welfare (2019-2021). This survey too found that more Indians drink to get drunk than people in the rest of the world.

Across various states in India, the proportion among consumers of alcohol who are alcohol dependent ranged between 4.7% and 48.3%. At the national level, this figure is 18.5%. More than 40% of alcohol users drink alcohol in a regular, dependent manner in the following places: Puducherry, Punjab, Andhra Pradesh and Karnataka. These places also have the largest numbers of persons with medical consequences of alcoholism like cirrhosis and cancers of the gastro-intestinal system.

85.4% of all Indians are teetotallers and another 9.4% of Indians drink sometimes, are not dependent and have no health or family problems attributed to drinking. 5.2% of all Indians are problem users in the sense that they are either dependent on alcohol or alcohol use by them has led to medical, social and personal problems like cirrhosis of the liver, violent outbursts, job loss and domestic violence. The fact that the vast majority of Indians (94.8%) are either teetotallers or drink sensibly and only a minority fall into the problem drinker category is important because it holds true for *all* drugs everywhere in the world. Both cross-sectionally and historically, a vast majority of people do not take a drug excessively even when it is available like alcohol is in most of India. And a vast majority of people who use a drug use it responsibly and are not harmed by it. Non-addicted users vastly outnumber addicted users.

This does not convey in any way that alcoholism or drug addiction are not an urgent public health issue but it helps us to understand that notwithstanding the moral outrage, carelessly spewed figures need a more objective look so that specific health services can be planned and a sane social response provided to those who need them.

If we juxtapose the national figures pertaining to alcohol use against the figures pertaining to Punjab we can see that presently Punjab has cause for concern. As far as the percentage of people who consumed alcohol in the previous one year is concerned, Punjab is at number three among all states. States with high prevalence of alcohol use in India are Chhattisgarh (35.6%), Tripura (34.7%), Punjab (28.5%), Arunachal Pradesh (28%) and Goa (28%) against the national average of 14.6%.

According to the National Family Health Survey conducted by the Union Ministry of Health and Family Welfare (2019-2021), alcohol consumption, both in men and women is more prevalent in the rural than in the urban population. It is also more common in Scheduled Tribes than in any other caste/ tribe groups. States with the highest prevalence of alcohol dependence as distinct from casual use of alcohol are Tripura (13.7%), Arunachal Pradesh (7.2%), Chhattisgarh, Punjab and Andhra Pradesh (around 6% each) against the national average of 2.7%. A person may not be an alcoholic but still may have run into issues because of an occasional bout of drinking. Thus, 4.5% of people in Punjab have been harmed by alcohol (health issues, fights, accidents, etc.) without being dependent on it, against the national average of 2.5%.

The most worrying part of the survey was that Punjab topped the list of all states as far as drinking by minors is concerned. 6% of minors had used alcohol in the previous one year at least once as compared to the national average of 1.3%. The reason in all probability is social acceptance and tolerance for alcohol in general.

Popular Punjabi music videos unabashedly romanticise alcohol and intoxicants. Sample this, *'Je tu peg* vodka *da, munda* liquid *feem kude.*' (Lassie, if you consider yourself a peg of vodka, I am liquid opium) and '*O kudi nachdi ae* vodka *de* peg *vargi, Chit kare ohnu gat gat pee jaavan.*' (She dances like a glass of vodka, I crave to gulp her down). Songs like these are played on loop at weddings and other social functions with youngsters dancing merrily to the peppy tunes.

The legal drinking age in Punjab is twenty-five years. In many states, it is twenty-one or eighteen. However, the legal age does not seem to matter in India since the actual verification of the age of buyers who go to purchase a drink at retail outlets or in restaurants is lackadaisical. Many of my patients suffering from alcoholism send their minor sons or minor servants to buy liquor for them, and they are often able to buy large supplies although they clearly look much younger than twenty-five. This probably holds true for most of India.

Tobacco

Tobacco was not included in this National Survey but the Global Adult Tobacco Survey India Factsheet of 2016-17 reports that in India, 8.6 % of adults (men-15.2 %, women-1.7%) smoke tobacco daily, while 18.2% of adults chew it daily (men-25.1%, women-11.1%). It seems a fairly large number of women are daily users of tobacco, but prefer to chew it or just keep it in their mouths than smoke because of restrictions at the workplace and social stigma in general.

This mode of smokeless consumption of tobacco is particularly important in Punjab because the majority of the population is Sikh and while the tenets of Sikhism prohibit the use of all intoxicants, smoking is looked upon as particularly abhorrent. This makes some Sikhs resort to chewing tobacco instead of smoking to escape religious exclusion!

Cannabis

In India, cannabis is commonly used as bhang, which is legally available in some states. The other two preparations which are stronger are ganja and charas—both of which are illegal across the country under the NDPS Act like heroin and other illicit drugs. Even consumption is a jailable offence

Bhang, ganja and charas are derived from the same plant. Charas or hashish is made from the resin of the plant (Cannabis sativa or Cannabis indica). Ganja is a Sanskrit word and corresponds most approximately to weed or marijuana of the West and is extracted from flowering tops of the plant. Bhang, ganja and charas, in that order, have increasing percentage of tetra-hydro cannabinol (THC) content which is the active agent of cannabis.

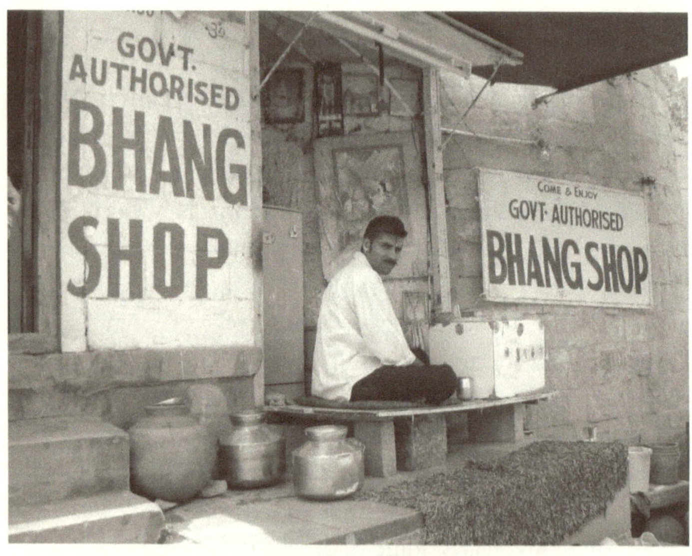

Government approved bhang shop in Jaisalmer, Rajasthan.
(Photo: Tom Maisey, *Wikimedia Commons*)

Bhang is the mildest of these three commonly used cannabis preparations. It is made from the leaves and seeds of the plant and is mostly ingested. It is eaten in snacks like fritters and added to *lassi* (drink made from yoghurt or buttermilk). Charas and ganja are mostly smoked. However, after weed has been liberalized in many countries entrepreneurs have come up with various edibles containing ganja too.

To prepare bhang, leaves of the plant Cannabis indica are ground into a paste which can be added to food items. To prepare a beverage, it is mixed with milk and filtered, then often flavoured with sugar, fruit and various spices.

The 1961 international treaty, the Single Convention on Narcotic Drugs, initially classed all cannabis class of drugs with hard drugs like opioids and cocaine. During the negotiations, the Indian delegation opposed this categorization, citing the use of bhang as part of our cultural tradition and a component of religious ceremonies of the majority Hindu religion. The suggestion was accepted. This allowed India to not just legally carry on the tradition of large-scale consumption of bhang during the festivals of Holi and Shivratri but also provided persons like manual labourers and farm workers the use of a cheap and relatively safe intoxicant. Bhang is available in government approved outlets in many states of North and East India.

2.83% of Indians aged 10-75 years (3.1 crore individuals) are current users of one of these three cannabis products. More people use bhang (2%) than charas/ganja (1.2%). There is a preponderance of men among consumers of cannabis. In India, users of cannabis outnumber users of opioids (2.83 vs 2.03% of the population)

In general, the trend in most Indian states is a higher prevalence of intake of bhang as compared to the stronger varieties like ganja or charas. However, the reverse trend is visible in some of the eastern and Northeastern states like West Bengal, Bihar, Sikkim, Mizoram, Nagaland and Meghalaya. Here, the illegal cannabis products, ganja or charas, are used by a larger proportion of people as compared to bhang.

The proportion of people with problematic cannabis use is modest. At the national level, only one in eleven cannabis users suffers from cannabis dependence. However, there is a substantial difference between bhang and ganja/charas in terms of dependent use and addiction. While just about one in sixteen users of bhang were dependent on cannabis, this figure was one in seven in the case of ganja/charas users. Ganja and charas are stronger cannabis preparations than bhang. States with high cannabis use are Uttar Pradesh, Punjab, Sikkim, Chhattisgarh and Delhi.

Over the decades, since the advent of the Green Revolution, a large number of people from eastern UP and Bihar have been going to Punjab, particularly during harvest time, to work as agricultural labourers. Many of them have stayed back there, learned the language, branched into other occupations like small businesses and construction-related activities and have been assimilated into Punjabi society. Use of cannabis is an intrinsic part of that sub-culture. One reason for Punjab figuring unexpectedly high on the cannabis charts is this immigrant population.

However, cannabis users do not show up in the clinics because it does not cause medical complications or organ damage and when stopped, there is no significant withdrawal. Usually, psychiatrists get to see patients with cannabis use the day after either Holi or Shivratri when some men from eastern UP or Bihar land up at their clinics with acute psychotic symptoms after an excessive celebratory intake of bhang. However, such psychotic episodes are short and clear up quickly even without treatment.

There is a recent trend of smoking weed among the youth living in metropolitan cities in India. In Punjab too, larger urban centres like Ludhiana and Mohali are showing increasing numbers of youngsters using marijuana, which starts as a peer-influenced fad to 'look cool'. Typically, at large parties, after some drinking, small groups of youngsters branch off to rooms to 'smoke up'.

Opioids

If we compare the usage of the three most common categories of intoxicants in the surveys done in 2004 (UNODOC, 2004) and in 2019 (National Magnitude Survey, 2019), while alcohol use seems to have been stable over the last fifteen years, cannabis use has increased by roughly one-and-a-half times, while the use of opioid drugs has increased three to four times.

Although the terms opioids and opiates are often used interchangeably, they are not synonymous:

The term opioid is all-inclusive and refers to all natural, semisynthetic and synthetic opioids. All these drugs act like opium and act on opioid receptors. These include:

a) opium and morphine which are natural products from the poppy of the plant Papaver somniferum.

b) heroin, which is modified from morphine in the laboratory by a simple chemical process.

c) a large number of synthetic pain-relieving medications like Tramadol, Dextropropoxyphene, Oxycodone, Hydrocodone, Fentanyl and Carfentanil—all of which are synthesized from scratch in the laboratory without needing any plant product. The number of such laboratory analogues has been increasing over the years as has been their potency.

The term *opiate* refers only to natural opioids derived directly from the plant Papaver somniferum such as opium, morphine and Codeine. While all opiates are opioids, all opioids are not opiates.

All of these drugs fall under the rubric of narcotic analgesics and are also used legitimately on medical advice for relief from severe pain after injuries or surgery, in terminal stages of cancer, when pain is severe and addiction is not the most important concern. It is also used to alleviate other painful conditions where routine pain relievers like Ibuprofen and Paracetamol do not work. All of the opioids also have cough suppressant actions like the parent drug opium. Codeine has historically been a component of many brands of cough syrups till most countries prohibited adding Codeine to them because of its addictive properties. Many opioids are used as injections in addition to their oral or nasal spray route and as skin patches. Certain select opioids like Methadone and Buprenorphine are used to treat patients suffering from heroin and opium addictions.

In 2004, the most common opioid used in India was crude plant-based opium, either as gum opium or poppy husk which is milder and has to be taken in a larger quantity for the same effect, followed by pharmaceutical opioids and heroin in the third place. By 2019, that order had been reversed with Indians' most preferred opioid drug being heroin, followed by pharmaceutical opioids and then opium. The shift from natural to laboratory produced opioid drugs has been clear and rapid. While opium is ingested, heroin is either ingested or snorted. Smoking is much less common. Pharmaceutical opioids come as oral preparations and as injections. Morphine is used only in injectable form.

The National Survey of 2019 has reported that 2.1% of all Indians have used opioids in the last one year for recreational purposes. It is a small proportion but adds up to about 2.5 crore individuals in absolute numbers.

4% of Indian males and 0.2% of females are opioid users. 1.8% of all minors in India between 10-18 years of age have taken an opioid drug in the last one year. 0.7% of all Indians have had medical, social, legal, occupational or family problems as a direct consequence of opioid use although all of them are not addicted. 0.26% of Indians are opioid dependent.

Out of the 99 lakh male problem users, 63 lakh use heroin, 25 lakh use prescription opioids, and 11 lakh use opium. The problem users/all users ratio is highest for heroin (1/2) followed by prescription opioids (1/4) and is the least for opium (1/5).

Opium, the oldest opioid, is thus the least commonly used opioid sub-category in modern times and has the lowest proportion of harmful or dependent users. These findings highlight the differences in the addictive property of different opioids. Harmful or dependent pattern was observed in half of all heroin users as compared to just one-fifth of opium users. These figures strongly support the argument by old timers that it is only the new synthetic and semisynthetic opioids, which are a problem, and not as much the opium which people were using in earlier decades.

In terms of percentage of population with problem use of opioids which needs treatment and help, the states at the top are Mizoram-6.9, Nagaland-6.5, Arunachal Pradesh-5.7, Sikkim-5.1, Manipur-4.0, Punjab-2.8, Haryana-2.5 and Delhi-2.3.

In general, the prevalence of opioid use in the northeast and northwest regions of India is higher compared to other regions. This geographical distribution in India of opioid use with higher concentration in the northeast and northwest was first reported in a 1928 publication by Chopra & Chopra.

There are geopolitical reasons for the worst affected states being in two opposite corners of the country. While the Northeastern states which are most affected have a border with Myanmar, the second highest illicit opium producing country in the world, the Northwestern states of Punjab, Haryana and Jammu & Kashmir share a border with Pakistan, the mountainous areas of which along with that of Afghanistan and Iran constitute the Golden Crescent, the highest opium producing region in the world.

Inhalants

Inhalant abuse (also known as volatile substance abuse, solvent abuse, snorting, huffing and bagging) is the deliberate inhalation of vapours of a volatile substance to achieve an altered mental state. Inhalant abuse is a serious and under-reported internationally prevalent disorder.

Inhalant abuse is the only category of addiction where the majority of sufferers are not adults but children. Most of these children are from poor and marginalized communities or from broken homes with a history of abuse. Many of them work at petrol stations or parking lots in cities where they sniff petrol from tanks of scooters and cars. Some work as assistants to house painters and sniff thinner fluid. Others who work as domestic servants sniff acetone, which is used as nail polish remover. Inhalant abuse of kerosene, petrol, gasoline and typewriter correction fluid have also been reported. Some of these children whose work involves polishing shoes develop addiction to boot polish vapours and they sniff polish repeatedly.

Naphthalene or mothballs, a commonly used substance in households and freely available in the market is an uncommon source of inhalant abuse, which may lead to severe medical complications.

Being legal, easily available, cheap, with faster onset of action because of the inhalation route and the capacity to give a regular high make inhalants a dangerous substance of abuse especially among the very young in cities and towns. Chronic use leads to severe anaemia. Resultant lack of oxygen to the brain, pneumonia and aspiration of vomitus can lead to death of children.

0.70% of Indians are current users of inhalant products. Prevalence in the adult population is 0.58% while the prevalence among children and adolescents is twice as much at 1.17%. One-fifth are addicted or are otherwise problem users. States with high population of children needing help for inhalant use are Uttar Pradesh, Madhya Pradesh, Maharashtra, Delhi and Haryana.

Sedatives

1.08% of people in India use sedatives without a prescription out of which one-tenth are dependent on these. Most of these are benzodiazepines, which are used by doctors for treating anxiety, panic attacks and psychosomatic conditions. Many patients continue to take them for years in small doses to fall asleep without suffering any apparent adverse effects. But these sedatives give rise to dependence and cannot and should not be stopped suddenly.

While mostly harmless as long as the dose is small, these can worsen memory problems in older patients.

Cocaine

Cocaine is a stimulant drug while alcohol and opioids are nervous system depressants. Unlike the American continent and some parts of Europe, cocaine is *not* a popular drug of addiction in India. Only a miniscule proportion—0.10% of Indians have in the previous one year used cocaine out of which only 0.02% are problem users. For Punjab, the figures are 0.66% and 0.20%. Arunachal Pradesh with 3.01% and 0.89% is the highest cocaine using state in India.

Amphetamines and MDMA or Ecstasy

These synthetic stimulant drugs have been historically used by militaries to counter fatigue and sleep and to improve concentration and by students to stay up late to prepare for their examinations. The only legitimate medical use of amphetamines is to treat attention deficit disorder (ADD) in children.

These are sometimes used as a recreational drug—alone or in combination. Amphetamines are addictive when high doses are taken for a long duration and can produce a typical paranoid reaction in which the person is excited, talks in a 'flighty' manner and is paranoid. Just 0.18% of people in India have used amphetamine type of drugs.

Ecstasy, another stimulant drug, is used worldwide as a recreational and party drug. It is sought out for its effects of increased energy, empathy, elation and heightened sensations. Whenever one reads of the police raiding a rave party in a farmhouse in the suburbs of a metropolis, one of the common drugs being used there is Ecstasy. Only 0.18% Indians have used Ecstasy in the recent past and 0.06% are problem users. Most of such use is limited to large cities. For Punjab, the figures are 0.64% and 0.24%.

All stimulant drugs including cocaine, amphetamines and Ecstasy are far less commonly used in India than in the US or Europe. The reasons for this differential preference are not clear yet.

Hallucinogens

This group of drugs, even in small doses, causes hallucinations, which are mostly visual involving the person 'seeing' things that are actually not there and sometimes also 'hearing' voices with startling clarity. These drugs provide what is called an alternate experience and are used as recreational drugs, often in groups or at parties. The most commonly used drug in this group is LSD.

Indians do not use these drugs commonly and most users like Ecstasy users are part of an urban culture limited to metropolitan cities. States with sizeable numbers of hallucinogen users are Maharashtra (six lakhs), Telangana (two lakhs), Kerala (one lakh) and Delhi (63,000). The National Survey mentions no figures for Punjab.

The stimulant drugs, Ecstasy and the hallucinogen group of drugs are not a public health concern in India although the drug enforcement authorities continue to be disproportionately interested in these. Observers have criticized the narcotic authorities' frequent high-profile 'busts' of rave parties under the glare of television cameras, detaining hundreds, many of them tourists, in police stations for weeks for mere consumption.

Persons Who Inject Drugs

Most of the persons who inject drugs inject heroin, or much less commonly, pain reliever opioids, to experience a quicker and stronger effect. The drug is injected into a vein by the person himself or by a peer with addiction. A much smaller number of persons inject sedatives.

Persons who inject drugs are a special public health concern because needles are often shared, and this leads to the spread of serious—and unless treated, fatal infections—like HIV, Hepatitis-B and Hepatitis-C. The other cause for concern is that persons with addiction, because of the erratic quality of heroin sold by smugglers, sometimes unwittingly inject an excessive dose resulting in sudden death, which is often called overdosage death (OD) in the press.

India has 8.5 lakh persons who inject drugs. States with the highest concentration of injectable drug users are as follows:

1. Delhi—population 1.9 crores; number of injectable drug users 87,000

2. Punjab—population 2.8 crores; number of injectable drug users 88,000

3. Northeastern states—population of eight states—4.6 crores; injectable drug users 1.5 lakh

4. Haryana—population 2.5 crores; number of injectable drug users 55,000

Since injectable drug users mostly inject opioid drugs, the geographical distribution of 'injectors' is the same as that of opioid users by the oral, nasal or smoking route. i.e., the northwest and the northeast of the country have the highest figures. 49% of intravenous drug users in Punjab have Hepatitis-C as a result of sharing needles, leading to a serious public health crisis. On the other hand, just 3% of people in Punjab who do not take drugs have Hepatitis-C.

Many countries in the world have reduced the prevalence of Hepatitis-C through awareness campaigns and by providing fresh syringes to addicts at selected spots in cities and by distributing syringes in the community hotspots where there is a concentration of persons with drug addiction.

~

Historically, drug addiction has been considered a predominantly male problem. However, this gender difference has been narrowing over the last decades. While alcohol, cannabis and smoking are still a lot more frequent among men, the gender differences in stimulants and prescription opiates dependence seem to have lessened in western countries. The overall male preponderance has been explained by citing the reason that women find it more difficult to access drugs. Different societal role expectations for men and women and drug use being more stigmatising for women in more traditional societies is another reason. Pregnancy and child rearing are deterrents too.

While women use drugs less frequently, they are more likely than men to develop addiction and other harmful effects because of physiological reasons. Women metabolise alcohol slower than men and because of this they are more likely to become intoxicated with the same amount of alcohol. There is also some evidence that both the ovarian hormones, oestrogen and progesterone, cross the blood-brain barrier and affect the brain centres involved in addiction. In some studies, women were found to drink more during the pre-menstrual phase and women with pre-menstrual syndrome (PMS) drank more than those who did not have PMS.

While a higher number of men initiate drug use to induce euphoria, women use drugs more commonly to alleviate pre-existing mental health problems like stress, depression or anxiety. This 'self-medication' among female users with the hope of feeling less depressed or anxious leads to a habit, which is more difficult to quit.

In India, according to the report of the National Survey of 2019, 'substance use exists in all the population groups, but adult men bear the brunt of substance use disorders.' Thus, while 27.3% of Indian men used alcohol just 1.6% of Indian women did which means that in India, for every one woman who drinks, there are seventeen men who drink.

For cannabis, the percentage of users in India are 5% of

men and 0.6% of all women. For opioid drugs like heroin and opium, the figures are 4% and 0.2% for men and women. Having a partner who is addicted to drugs, being subjected to domestic violence and being involved in peddling drugs increase the chances of addiction in women.

These gender differences become even more stark when it comes to seeking treatment for drug addiction. Most psychiatrists will be able to count on their fingers the number of female patients they have treated for addiction in the last one year. The reason for this scarcity of women in treatment (in addition to the actual numbers being low), is the stigma being much worse for women. While society gives a lot of leeway to men when it comes to the use of intoxicants, it expects women to stay stone cold sober making it difficult for them to seek treatment.

In recent years, there have been some attempts on the part of the government at starting exclusive treatment facilities for women with substance use problems. However, in two years, Navjeevan at Kapurthala—the Punjab government's only exclusive rehab facility for women in the state, registered seventy clients while 10,000 male drug users were registered in the Kapurthala government facility alone (*The Tribune*, June 3, 2019).

CHAPTER 7

Saving Young Lives, Preventing Overdosage Deaths

Unlike alcohol and tobacco, opioid drugs do not cause any serious medical illness other than addiction. Injections of heroin in pure, uncontaminated form in steady and small doses, do not cause organ damage or death. However, if syringes and needles are shared among persons with addiction, it can lead to the spread of HIV or Hepatitis-C infections from one user to another. If left untreated, HIV can result in death by compromising the immune system of the host and inviting fatal opportunistic infections. In the case of untreated Hepatitis-C, death occurs because of liver damage. However, these are not sudden deaths and often there is a period of years between contracting the infection and death.

The only way medically pure heroin can lead to sudden death is by an overdosage in which case, unless the person is rescued and treated right away, he can die in a matter of minutes due to respiratory failure. Most of these deaths are 'young deaths'. Overdosage deaths occur most commonly in persons who inject and sometimes among those who smoke heroin. It is much less common in addicts who use heroin by snorting because the required concentration is not reached that quickly and the user would become sedated before respiratory knockout can occur, and hence, would have stopped snorting.

According to the WHO factsheet of 2021, about 500,000 deaths are attributable to drug use worldwide annually. More than 70% of these are related to opioids, with more than 30% caused by overdose. There are effective treatment interventions for opioid dependence that can decrease the risk of overdose, yet, less than 10% of people who need such treatment is receiving it.

In the USA, according to a report by the National Institute of Drug Abuse, drug overdose deaths rose from 16,849 in 1999 to 70,237 in 2017. In the ten years prior to 2017, the number of overdose deaths doubled in the country.

Collating the latest available death certificate data, the Center for Disease Control and Prevention estimated that 100,300 Americans died of drug overdoses from May 2020 to April 2021, crossing the 100,000 per year mark for the first time. US President Joe Biden called it 'a tragic milestone' in a speech as government officials persuaded Congress to sanction billions of dollars more to address the problem. This figure included deaths from heroin, a new synthetic pain reliever fentanyl, older prescription pain relievers and other illicit drugs. Opioid overdosage deaths now kill more people in the USA each year than AIDS did in its most destructive phase and more people each year than the total number of American soldiers who died in the twenty years of the Vietnam War.

Most overdosage deaths are accidental and not suicidal. Hardly ever is there an intention to die. Most persons with addiction are quite familiar with the way their body responds to a drug because of having used it for a long time and are unlikely to make a mistake, other things remaining constant. But other things do *not* remain constant. There are important reasons for this. The most significant is that all these drugs are illegal and hence sold in secrecy. Because of the illicit nature of business, there is no question of customers being able to demand quality as their right.

The heroin sold in the city lanes and on the canal bridges in the villages of Punjab is very different in terms of quality from what a makeshift laboratory in rural Afghanistan would have sold to a Taliban cartel a month back. And there are multiple middlemen involved in the long journey of the drug as it crosses two international borders and reaches the consumer. The illegality of all these transactions is an implicit guarantee that none of those middlemen can be held responsible for the quality. During these multiple transactions, each seller down the line adulterates it a bit to make extra money, taking out a small amount of the drug and adding some benign white powder of the right consistency like sugar, starch, powdered milk or talcum powder to make up for the bulk and the weight. This process is called 'cutting'. By the time it reaches the user it could be 4% or 60% heroin. And no quality control is possible because the product is illegal to start with and consumer protection laws do not apply. In fact, the mere mention of the idea would raise a laugh.

What if every time you picked up a bottle of whiskey, you had no idea if it contained 4% alcohol or 40%? Chances are that sooner or later you will end up badly drunk or even unconscious. But this would not happen because alcohol is legal, quality control can be enforced, and the seller hauled up. Heroin being illegal also means that the person with addiction who takes the drug does it in secrecy to avoid being seen by both the family as well as the police. As a result, the addict ends up in deserted parks, old ruins or abandoned buildings to 'shoot up' and when overdosage occurs nobody can spot the person for hours or often for days.

Let us imagine a young man who in the previous weeks has been injecting 5 ml of a white powder mixed with distilled water, which contains only 10% of active heroin to get a certain high he is used to. Suppose the new supply that he gets one morning happens to contain 30% of heroin without his knowledge and he injects the same 5 ml as usual. This is three times what his system is used to. There is a high chance he will die of an overdosage. This utter lack of predictability about the quality of heroin is the most common cause of overdosage deaths. *The person dies not because he is looking for a higher level of intoxication but because he is looking for the same level of intoxication.*

However, even in the murky world of opioid selling and buying, cartels are conscious that if the consumers do not get a 'high' they will end up either looking for a different vendor in the next town or queue up at de-addiction centres for treatment. Nobody in the sellers' chain wants that. Here comes the process of cutting not with something bland and inert but with something stronger and much cheaper than heroin. In recent years, many opioid drugs have been synthesized in laboratories which fit these two requirements. The latest of these is Fentanyl. It is far more powerful and much cheaper to produce than heroin, which is derived from opium and tweaked in a lab. Fentanyl can be synthesized in the laboratory from scratch.

Fentanyl is often added at the point of manufacture of heroin by cartels, particularly during times of shortage of heroin. Different synthetic variants of Fentanyl, with wildly varying potency, turn up unpredictably in different locations around the world. Some drugs are so new they have not even been declared illegal and some, like Carfentanil, originally designed to tranquilize large animals, are extremely powerful—as much as

10,000 times stronger than morphine. It is this wildly fluctuating quality of heroin caused by cutting and adulterating, which is responsible for a large proportion of overdosage deaths.

Switzerland in the 1980s and 90s was one of the worst opioid addiction-affected countries in the world. But things changed when the drug policy was overhauled under a reformist woman President. Instead of jailing addicts who used heroin, the government itself started heroin clinics where heroin injections were given under medical supervision. As a result, the overdose deaths fell dramatically as did deaths due to HIV and Hepatitis-C.

Another cause of overdosage deaths is the treatment of opioid addiction and the period of abstinence after it. If addiction restarts after a period of 'staying clean', the chances of overdosage are more than what they would have been if the person had been using heroin continuously and not gone into treatment. This seems bizarre on the face of it but it is actually not. Abstinence for some weeks or months results in the person's body losing the tolerance to heroin, which had been built up over time while he was using the drug. And if he happens to relapse and take the drug again, he is likely to take the same dose which he was taking earlier just before the treatment. His body will not be able to tolerate that dose now because of 'breaking' of tolerance. This is just like a person who drinks after a very long interval and feels more drunk than at the time when he was drinking regularly. Only, this is far more dangerous.

In a 2003 study titled 'Loss of Tolerance and Overdose Mortality after Inpatient Opiate Detoxification,' published in the *British Medical Journal*, the authors concluded: 'Patients who "successfully" completed inpatient detoxification were more likely than other patients to have died within a year. No patient who failed to complete detoxification died. The clustering of the deaths from overdose in the group of patients who had successfully completed treatment is counterintuitive and illogical—unless it derives from loss of tolerance and consequent unpredictability of resumed heroin use...A similar increase in mortality among *released* prisoners who were formerly opiate addicts has been attributed to loss of tolerance and erroneous judgment of the dose when they returned to opiate use.'

Before any runaway conclusions are drawn, to put things in proper perspective, the mortality rate of opiate addicts for same age groups is ten times more than that of non-addicts in many countries even when deaths because of HIV/AIDS as a result of shared syringes, are excluded. The treatment of addiction reduces this mortality rate several times. *Except* transiently in this specific situation of treatment-induced abstinence, followed by relapse. The reason is that while tolerance of the body to heroin is lost, craving for it may not have decreased proportionately, leading to a relapse and a keenness to take the same dose as the person had been taking before treatment.

The answer to this dilemma clearly lies in making this information a part of the treatment process to be given at an appropriate time in a delicate manner. Here, the problem most of the time is not the patient but the treating team which might be painting the situation in black and white by not discussing relapse at all. In their view, the whole purpose of the treatment is to not to have a relapse, and so 'why put the idea in the patient's mind?' The field of de-addiction treatment is full of such moralistic and unrealistic notions and society's beliefs often infect even some of those who treat the patients, as we will see when we look into the debate between the 'harm reduction' versus the 'abstinence' approaches of treatment.

However, when it is a question of preventing overdosage

deaths, it is vital that the treatment process is transparent rather than romantic. This would essentially involve a frank discussion about the reality that relapses unfortunately do occur and that a period of abstinence leads to breaking down of tolerance and if the usual dose is taken after it, it might amount to a fatal overdosage. There is no evidence at all in scientific literature to prove that imparting this lifesaving information increases the chances of relapse just as there is no evidence to prove that asking a depressed patient about the presence of suicidal ideas increases the chances of suicide by 'putting the idea of suicide' into the person's head.

A future relapse should be treated as a realistic possibility and discussed in a pragmatic manner, covering all its ramifications. This discussion between the psychiatrist and the patient is essential. There is no room here for paternalism or for morality. The problem with the proverbial elephant in the room is that it does not go away if you ignore it.

Opiate overdosage is eminently reversible if treated in time with an intravenous injection of Naloxone, an opiate antagonist. The challenge is that it must be done right away because what an opiate overdosage does is to suppress the respiratory centre in the brain. Time is of the essence. All emergency departments in hospitals and all de-addiction centres have the antidote but the difficulty is that the patient is rarely brought there in time. If the patient gets there in time, the recovery is miraculous. Recently, Naloxone sprays have also become available, which can be administered by anyone with a minimum amount of training. Unfortunately, many of the ambulance services in India do not have Naloxone injections on board.

Since many persons with addiction are found behind locked doors after an overdosage, the fire department is the first responder to reach them in some countries such as the USA.

The fire fighters are trained in diagnosing heroin overdosage and carry Naloxone injections and Naloxone nasal sprays.

Heroin(e) (2017), an American movie which was nominated for the best documentary at the Academy Awards comes to mind. It documents the community's integrated response to the overdose crisis in the town of Huntington, West Virginia, where the overdose rate is ten times the US average. The focus is on three women professionals of the community: Huntington Fire Chief Jan Rader who treats overdose victims along with other first responders; Cabell County Judge Patricia Keller, who heads the drug court; and Necia Freeman of Brown Bag Ministry, who delivers food to women who resort to prostitution to support their addictions.

The documentary clearly explains the use of Naloxone to treat overdose victims and looks at the psychological toll on the county's first responders who handle dozens of overdoses a month. It follows first responders as they respond to calls, including one instance where a woman is revived at the counter of a convenience store while customers continue to shop ten feet away. There are dozens of interviews with people who were addicted and are in recovery, who discuss the effects of drugs on their lives and their efforts to recover from addiction.

All policy makers in the field of de-addiction services in India, particularly in Punjab and in the Northeast would do well to watch *Heroine* from the point of view of co-opting community resources like the fire department and training fire fighters to diagnose and treat overdosage at site. In Punjab, there is no institutionalized mechanism for gathering and disseminating information about overdosage deaths. Drug addiction has been used as a political tool to beat up the government in power by successive opposition parties, who make their own wild promises to wipe off the scourge of addiction from Punjab for good, once *they* come to power. And when they do come to power, every piece of news of an overdosage death—because of its dramatic nature and high visibility—is construed as a reminder that they failed. It does not have to be perceived that way, but it is. Hence, such data is suppressed by the new government.

It is crucial to track the number of overdosage deaths systematically so that preventive measures can be organized. If data is suppressed the response would be flawed. Because of the terrible stigma surrounding overdosage deaths families too add to the problem by not reporting such deaths.

Since the issue has been so deeply politicized, governments are not keen to have a separate institutional mechanism to monitor overdosage deaths or even to a have a separate OD management unit either at the state or district level. And when forced to part with figures either in response to questions in the Legislative Assembly or queries under the right to information (RTI) act, the figures available are disjointed, contradictory and are not amenable to being converted into graphs, which clearly show the increase or decrease in numbers over a period of time.

The Tribune of March 29, 2019 reported, 'Even as the government has been denying reports related to deaths due to drug overdose, information procured under the RTI from the state police has confirmed that ninety-five youths had lost their lives in such cases last year, averaging eight per month. The media had widely reported drug-related deaths in June and July last year, but the state government remained evasive on the issue for several months. The government's contrasting stand was witnessed in the last Assembly session too, when initially Health Minister Brahm Mahindra said there were just two such deaths and later, in reply to a question in the House, he revealed that chemical examination confirmed fifty-six drug deaths in 2018-19 and eleven in 2017-18.'

The fact is that even the figures given out by the government are likely to be a gross underestimate because families do not report such deaths when the deaths occur at home, or when a family member is the first person to reach the site, because of both the social stigma and the fear of intensive police questioning.

In June and July of 2018 when there was a spike in the number of overdosage deaths reported in the press, the state government reacted in panic with a slew of baffling measures. The government's first action was that deputy commissioners of several districts in Punjab issued orders to ban the sale of hypodermic syringes without a doctor's prescription.

The order was met with a vociferous reaction from public health experts from all over the country. They pointed out that this was a regressive, even dangerous step because it would actually push desperate addicts into a corner and force them to share syringes repeatedly to conserve them and would lead to an epidemic of Hepatitis-C and HIV in Punjab (*The Indian Express*, July 8, 2018).

'By banning syringes, you want to make needles and syringes difficult to access. But the problem is you are putting people at risk. When the same needle and syringe will be shared by different people due to shortage, there is a high risk that deadly diseases like HIV could be transmitted,' Dr Atul Ambekar of the National Drug Dependence Treatment Centre told *The Indian Express*.

It was pointed out that while European governments were sending free syringes in dedicated vans to persons with addiction in areas where drug addiction was common, the Punjab government had passed this regressive, counter-intuitive measure. This was indeed a kneejerk reaction and not a well-conceived plan at all. Nobody seemed to have given a thought to the fate of diabetes patients who administer insulin injections to themselves several times a day. These patients far outnumbered drug addicts and if they had to go back to their doctors for prescriptions for syringes, life would be so much harder for them.

Chemists and pharmacists who had already been complaining about harassment and repeated inspections by drug inspectors saw red and declared that henceforth they would not stock or sell syringes *even on prescriptions* to avoid intrusive inspections. A public health expert pointed out the illegality of the order by reminding the authorities that the Drug and Cosmetic Act laid down that a doctor's prescription was essential for only a category of drugs, and syringes, by no stretch of the imagination, could be classified as drugs. All in all, it was quite a mess.

When the finger pointing began, the Department of Health backtracked claiming it had not been consulted by the district administrators but a government psychiatrist at Kapurthala in an interview to *The Indian Express* on July 8, 2018 asserted that the government's order was logical and the shortage of syringes would force persons with addiction to visit health facilities, 'We can then help by providing proper treatment' he reasoned, thus, grossly underestimating the intensity and urgency behind the craving of a person, who has been addicted to heroin and injects heroin several times a day. The fact is that when such patients do not get fresh syringes, they do not go to doctors for prescriptions for syringes. They either share syringes or rummage through garbage heaps and city parks for used syringes.

The order was quietly withdrawn later. However, a year-and-a-half down the line, out of fear, chemists still refused to sell syringes to young men. When a barely nineteen-year-old patient told me this, I asked him, 'How can they do it? The order was withdrawn and besides there are diabetics too who need syringes.'

The young man looked at me with a bitter smile, 'Do I look like a diabetic?'

So, even the withdrawn order, more than two years later, continued to cause damage because fearful pharmacists and chemists refused to sell syringes to all young men, because they thought it was better to be safe than sorry.

~

When persons with addiction are injecting drugs in pairs or in small groups, if one of them looks sleepy or unwell, a friend would rush him to the nearest hospital where a single injection of Naltrexone would revive him immediately in most cases. This was done despite the risk of being questioned and detained by the police for using illicit drugs. However, in 2018, in cases of overdosage deaths the police started arresting persons in whose presence the overdosage had happened, charging them with culpable homicide, which carries a sentence of ten years. This illogical policy continues resulting in co-addicts fleeing out of fear and leaving their friend to die at the first sign of overdosage unlike earlier, when they would have taken the person to a hospital and saved his life.

The government also announced the setting up of an advisory board to enable detention of drug smugglers for a year without trial. It recommended to the central government that death sentence should be accorded for peddlers and smugglers of illicit drugs (even first-time offenders). The NDPS Act already provides for death sentence for repeat offenders.

As is evident, the thrust of the state response was confined to more policing and even harsher punishments. There was no response along the lines of raising public awareness about the causes of overdosage deaths and educating people on how to save lives.

The emphasis should have been on training doctors, nurses, ambulance personnel, paramedics working in primary health centres and community health centres in diagnosing heroin overdosage, in giving injections of Naloxone or spray and doing CPR. The emphasis should have been on thinking out of the box and involving other departments like the fire department, panchayats and ASHA workers who are there in all villages, in a concerted effort to rescue and treat such patients.

It was also essential to ensure that Naloxone injections and Naloxone nasal sprays were available freely at these sites and with all these personnel. Since the injections are rarely used (but are lifesaving when used), it is important to periodically replace these with fresh supplies. The UNODC-WHO standards of care in 2019 laid down the principles of treatment of opioid addictions, one of which is handing over the antidote injection Naloxone to patients themselves along with instructions so that it can be used if required in an emergency. None of the above have been implemented.

CHAPTER 8

The Nature of Addiction

According to Dr Ronald D. Siegel, the need to periodically alter our wake consciousness is an instinctual need. It is the fourth instinct after food, sex and sleep. At the root of this drive, he says, is the motivation to feel 'different from normal, a holiday from reality'. Some people reach this state through travel, books, art, roller coasters, sport, religion, exploration, love, social contact or power. Others use intoxicants. 'It's the same motivation,' says Dr Siegel. 'We wouldn't live if we didn't seek to feel different.'

Since time immemorial human beings across the globe have felt this natural urge to feel different on a periodic or regular basis. Children discover the experience quite early when they playfully spin around at increasing speed till they feel a headrush. They do it despite the giddiness because the headrush is an unfamiliar and an exhilarating feeling. That is also why young girls play *kikli* in pairs, holding each other's hands and spinning around in circles, egged on by their friends to go faster, and at the height of spinning, shrieking in glee. The pituitary gland located at the bottom of the brain produces chemicals called endorphins, which make the spinning girls feel thrilled. Interestingly, endorphins have an action very similar to that of morphine. Like morphine and other opioids, endorphins reduce the perception of pain and trigger a happy and relaxed feeling. The word endorphin is a blend of 'endogenous' and 'morphine', meaning endorphins are morphine produced normally by the human body.

Ironically, if endorphins produced by your brain could be put in a vial, it would be a crime anywhere in the world to carry that vial in your pocket!

The biological ubiquity of the urge to feel intoxicated is supported by the large body of evidence available about many species of animals repeatedly ingesting certain plants, which contain intoxicating chemicals. This happens not accidentally but intentionally. Cats lunge at anything laced with catnip oil and then roll around playfully, purring, pawing and frisking about. Elephants in West Bengal get drunk on moonshine and go on a rampage often. Parrots nibble on poppy pods in Rajasthan and Madhya Pradesh and fly away in a daze. Farmers say opium has affected the genetic material of parrots over the generations and they are programmed to steal opium pods and eat them.

In his book, *Intoxication,* Dr Siegel notes that bees, after gorging on the numbing nectar of particular orchids, drop to the ground for a few minutes and then fly back for more. 'Birds poach on inebriating berries, then fly with carefree abandon. Cats eagerly sniff aromatic 'pleasure' plants, then play with imaginary objects. Cows look for special weeds with single-minded motivation and after chewing on them, some will twitch, shake and unsteadily walk back to the plants for more. Elephants purposely get drunk on fermented fruits. Snacking on magic mushrooms cause monkeys to sit with their heads on their hands in a posture reminiscent of Rodin's *The Thinker.* The pursuit of intoxication by animals seems as purposeless as it is passionate.'

According to Dr Siegel, history shows that people have always used intoxicants. From the beginning of civilization, people across the world have turned to plant-based drugs, alcohol and a variety of other mind-altering substances to feel intoxicated. In fact, this behaviour has as much force and persistence as that of our three basic drives for food, sleep and sex. Noah's Ark, Siegel writes, 'would have looked a lot like London on a Saturday night'.

~

Whether it is opium, cannabis, cocaine, tobacco or alcohol, exposure of mankind to plant-based drugs, which relieve pain and/or give pleasure through their action on the brain has been long and pervasive. These five primary drugs have been intimately intertwined with human existence for thousands of years and integrated into daily living. Over millennia, human beings and these plants have evolved in a co-dependent manner.

The fact that certain plants have tremendous medical uses has been known to human beings for long. Their recreational use has been a surprise, an exciting bonus of sorts, and the result of a long and intricate evolutionary process. There are certain active chemicals found in these plants, which affect the human brain; similar chemicals already exist naturally in the brain and are produced indigenously by the body. For example, while morphine produced by the opium plant is responsible for its remarkable pain relieving and euphoriant effects, endorphins with similar effects like morphine are produced naturally in our nervous systems. In the body, endorphins are produced as a reaction to pain but also as a reaction to vigorous physical exercise, resulting in the so-called 'runners' high'. Endorphins are also produced during pleasurable activities like sex, orgasm and eating delectable food (chocolates for instance, irrespective of the exact cocoa content).

Endorphins, in addition to their own euphoriant effect, increase the production of dopamine, the main pleasure chemical in the brain. Endorphins are also called 'endogenous opioids' to distinguish these from exogenous opioids produced outside the body by the poppy plant and in pharmaceutical factories. Our bodies, in this sense, are walking, talking narcotic factories, which happen to be legal.

Molecules of opioid drugs, whether endogenous or exogenous, produce all their effects on humans by locking on to tiny, customized and microscopic receptacles in the brains called opioid receptors. These receptacles are tailor-made reception centres to receive the body's self-produced endorphins, morphine from a poppy plant or a factory, and heroin coming from Afghanistan. There is no bias at work here.

~

The basic functional units of the nervous system are brain cells called neurons. The opioid receptors are present in some of these neurons. Neurons have a cell body and a long tail called axon, which connects with the next neuron down the line and so on. These chains of neurons convey signals with remarkable alacrity from and to other parts of the brain and from the brain to the rest of the body and back. A group of chemicals (neurotransmitters) facilitate the electrical impulse to jump from one neuron to the next across the short gap between the two. That is how different parts of the brain talk with one another and with the rest of the body. This is a two-way talk.

When a pin pricks your toe, an electrical impulse goes up along the relay of neurons, facilitated by neurotransmitters across the gaps, to the part of the brain which perceives pain.

The brain then sends back an order to the leg muscles to withdraw the foot from the pin. The whole process from the pin prick to the foot being pulled away takes a fraction of a millisecond.

Whenever a person takes opium or heroin, it enters his blood and then crosses the blood brain barrier into the brain. When it reaches the opioid receptors, messages go out to those parts of the brain whose function is to produce a feeling of euphoria and those parts deliver euphoria. The messages also simultaneously go to the parts of the brain, which increase the secretion of dopamine, the broad-spectrum pleasure chemical, making the person relaxed and happy.

Cannabis, the second plant-based intoxicant which is as old as opium and is like opium has been with human beings for thousands of years.

Cannabis is known as weed, bhang, charas, hashish, ganja, marijuana and by many other names in different parts of the world. Cannabis-based drugs produce their effects through the cannabinoid receptors in our bodies. Uncannily, cannabis-like chemicals are also normally produced in the human body just like endorphins and are called endocannabinoids.

The functions of endocannabinoids are to facilitate physical exercise, improve mood and memory, help in female reproduction, modulate response to stress and increase our sense of arousal during novel situations. Other than this, cannabinoid receptors mediate the effects of cannabis drugs like bhang, ganja, charas and marijuana if and when the individual happens to take them.

Not only does the human body produce its own cannabis but the brain also has custom-made micro-receiving sites with exact fit—a set of receptors to welcome cannabinoid molecules from outside the body just as it does for opioids.

A believer might conclude God made our bodies in such a manner so that if we wished to, we could use drugs. Either that or evolution over millions of years moulded our brains in this manner so that we could use recreational drugs. Just like evolution made a giraffe's neck longer so that it could reach the branches at a height. God or evolution, the believer may argue, did not want either the giraffe or homo sapiens to be content with the routinely available low hanging fruits!

While in the case of opium and of cannabis there is already a natural twin of each inside our body and also customized reception systems to welcome both drugs, the other drugs of recreation act through borrowed receptors in the brain, which normally have a different set of functions to perform. Thus, nicotine acts through cholinergic receptors, cocaine through dopamine receptors, alcohol through GABA receptors and LSD through serotonin receptors.

Opioid receptors are wired inside our brains in such a systematic manner that not just pain is relieved, but positive pleasure is generated through firing up of areas of the brain, increasing the levels of dopamine. Most of the other standard drugs routinely used for pain relief like Aspirin or Ibuprofen relieve pain without producing any bonus pleasure.

~

Not all drug use in the service of improving one's mood could be dysfunctional since the human body does exactly that on its own too even when there is no drug in sight for miles. Addiction is qualitatively very different from the 'judicious use' of drugs. It is not just about judicious use turning into excessive use— this is only one aspect. Additionally, the use of drugs is to the detriment of the organism because:

i) The drug is now causing functional or structural damage to the body.

ii) Drug use is compulsive in nature. The person cannot help taking it.

iii) The addicting substance (or behaviour) consumes one's mind space, making everything else—relationships, work and friends—insignificant and in the long run, altering one's life comprehensively. This quality of addiction is called *salience*.

iv) Because of its salience and compulsive nature, addiction progressively narrows down one's mind space and time for work and relationships with others including close family members.

Another hallmark of addiction is that even when a person is in the throes of the worst addiction, he *knows* that he should not be taking the drug, but he still does. It is as if an irresistible external force is at play. The mind is working at two levels, one at which the person is aware that he must not take the drug and another at which he decides to go ahead and take it.

Well-known English poet, critic and philosopher Samuel Taylor Coleridge was known to have been a regular user of opium. He used it as a relaxant, pain reliever, antidepressant and as a treatment for his numerous health concerns. He is said to have written his famous poem, *Kubla Khan; Or, A Vision in a Dream: A Fragment* under the effect of opium. However, at one point of time, he was so sick of his habit and so helpless in controlling it that he is said to have hired a few men to stop him from entering a pharmacy if he tried to buy opium, highlighting the fascination, the intense craving and the utter helplessness of a person with addiction.

Iconic Greek bard Homer in his epic poem, *Odyssey*, tells the story of the ten-year-long journey of Odysseus (also known as Ulysses)—the emperor of Ithaca, who was sailing home after the Trojan War. On the way, his ship has to sail past an island populated by Sirens. In Greek mythology, a Siren is a creature who is half-bird and half-woman and sings enchantingly. Sirens sit beside the ocean, combing their long golden hair and singing to passing sailors. Those who hear their song are bewitched by its sweetness and drawn to the Sirens' island like iron filings to a magnet. Ships which are thus drawn smash upon rocks which are sharp as spears, and sailors end up with the many victims of the Sirens in a meadow filled with skeletons.

However, Odysseus had been warned about the Sirens and did not trust himself to be able to resist their pull. But he was also keen to hear the famous song and still survive. So, he ordered his crew of sailors to seal their ears with beeswax to ensure they would not hear the song of the Sirens. He also ordered them to tie him firmly to the ship's mast. He is firmly tied, and his men have the beeswax in their ears when they row their ship alongside the Sirens' island. Then, Odysseus hears the magical song as it floats over the summertime waters. He longs to plunge into the waves and to swim to the island. Despite being aware of the risk, he strains against the bonds which bind him to the ship's mast. Scowling at his crew, he urges them to free him. To his crew, made deaf with beeswax for the time being, the Sirens seem like hungry monsters with vicious, crooked claws. The ship speeds forward and soon the song of the Sirens is a distant echo. Only then do the crew members stop rowing and unbind their grateful captain, who has now come to his senses.

Many manage to take drugs, get away with pleasure and escape pain and death. For others, it is as much of a tightrope walk as Odysseus hearing the enchanting song, being drawn to the fabled sirens and narrowly escaping doom. The insight into the overpowering nature of one's own addiction makes some people with addiction hand over important decision-making about their life and treatment to a friend or a loved one temporarily.

For most alcohol and drug users, this dilemma rarely arises. Of all the people who use substances, only some make the leap from controlled use to addiction. Even after repeated exposure to drugs, addiction is the *exception* not the rule. Nicotine is one of the most powerfully addictive substances known to mankind. Even then, only a portion of the young people who experiment with smoking for fun or to feel like adults or feel 'liberated' become addicted. But there is no way to foretell with surety who would and who would not. Despite current scientific advances, we will have to wait for evidence to be produced by research in the fields of genetics and social sciences to ascertain this.

Those Who Get Away with Pleasure without Getting Addicted

In India, despite the easy availability of alcohol, which is legally available in the whole country except in a few states, one out of seven persons out of the whole population between ten and seventy-five years of age drink even casually. Six out of seven Indians are teetotallers despite easy availability. Even among those who drink, 18% end up as alcoholics and the other 82% go through life drinking for pleasure without getting addicted to alcohol.

The proportion of persons who use drugs in India without getting addicted are as follows in the three most commonly used categories of drugs:

Alcohol — 72%

Opioid drugs — 87.4 %

Cannabis drugs — 91.2 %

The percentage of people who use opioids and cannabis are higher in Punjab than all-India figures but even in Punjab, the percentage of users who do not get addicted in spite of using opioids are approximately the same as in the rest of the country:

Alcohol — 69%
Opioid drugs — 87 %
Cannabis — 97 %

The Northeastern states of India have the highest usage of opioid drugs among all Indian states (14-25%). But there too, 85% of those who take opioids do not get addicted.

At a global level, the proportion of persons who get addicted to drugs out of all the persons who use drugs is about the same as in India. In the UNODC world drug report of 2019, it is recorded that 12.9% of persons who took 'illicit drugs' developed addiction.

In pointing out that only a small proportion of people who take drugs become addicted to usage, the aim is to understand addiction and not to make light of either the drug addiction situation in India or the world. The idea is also not to tell you to go ahead and take these drugs since 87% chances are that you will not get addicted. Never forget that there is a 13% chance that you will and this will change your life and that of your family for worse. It has to be emphasized that there is no way to predict whether a person would fall in the 'safe' category of 87% or in the catastrophic 13%.

Drug addiction is a serious and destructive disorder—particularly, opioid addiction, with the escalatory ladder going on to injectable use with disastrous consequences to the individual, the family and to society as a whole. And even with 13% of users of opioids becoming addicted to opioids, in absolute numbers, this translates to as many as 28 lakh persons in the country and 3.84 lakhs just in Punjab, which is a huge public health burden, apart from the human misery and productivity loss involved.

What are the attributes that differentiate the 13% of users of opioids who get 'hooked' and the 87% who take these drugs and do not get addicted? It is important to study these because it is in the differences between the attributes of these two groups—whether it is genetics, the environment, social factors and early childhood—that we are likely to find the true determinants of addiction.

Addiction is a Brain Disease

The current scientific view after decades of research is that drug addiction is not a bad habit, a personal failing or an immoral trait; it is a chronic, relapsing disease like hypertension, diabetes or rheumatoid arthritis. This by no means implies that certain persons are immune to addictions whatever they do and others are doomed to addictions whatever precautions they take. Every person with a genetic propensity to hypertension or diabetes does not manifest with the diseases. Others suffering from diabetes and hypertension may not have a family history of the diseases. There are many intervening variables which may influence the final outcome. The most significant of these is psychological trauma—particularly during the formative years.

As is true of other non-communicable chronic diseases, the 'medical model' of addiction does not exclude the fact that stress and unemployment or abusive relationships can be reasons for triggering and sustaining addiction. Therefore, correcting societal and family stressors are as important as medical treatment.

Consider this analogy: even though tuberculosis is clearly an infectious disease overall community management must include steps to ameliorate overcrowding and poverty because it is under these conditions that tuberculosis thrives. Creating better living conditions for people is as important as the medical treatment, which targets the tuberculosis germ. In the same manner, effective management of addictions by society cannot afford to exclude social and economic issues like the lack of jobs, which contribute to addiction.

Some may question the logic of the concept of addiction being an illness. Isn't addiction something the individual brings upon himself? Nobody forces him to take drugs. Why can't he stop taking them? To take them or not—isn't that a matter of free will? Such arguments are often put forward as if thinking along these lines is extremely logical. Except it is not so. Because both environmental factors like the availability of drugs and the dominance of choice operate only in the initial stages. When addiction sets in, biological factors take over. Very soon, it becomes less and less a matter of choice and more and more a matter of compulsion.

Often the dose of the drug needs to be increased for the person to get the same level of high. This is called tolerance. One needs three drinks after a while to feel the same level of relaxation, which earlier set in with two. Later on, the individual's body becomes dependent on the drug and not taking it produces withdrawal symptoms. In the case of opioids like heroin withdrawal is exceptionally distressing consisting of severe pains, watery eyes and nose and diarrhoea. In the case of alcohol too, if the person has been drinking large amounts (like one or two bottles of whiskey a day), withdrawal can be sudden and dramatic. After two days of not drinking, one starts having tremors and shakiness, becomes delirious and has vivid hallucinations of insects and tiny animals crawling all over one's body. This is called delirium tremens (DT) or 'the shakes'.

Coming back to the question: in addiction, is drug intake a compulsion because not taking it produces withdrawal symptoms? Does a person take the drug even when he does not want to because he fears the impending withdrawal? Both withdrawal and tolerance happen because the body has become dependent on the drug. Becoming physiologically dependent on the drug is normal after a certain time; all of us, depending on the nature of the drug can become dependent after taking it for weeks or months, even if we have a strong will and are not genetically prone to addiction.

The body can undergo withdrawal for some days even after abruptly stopping some of the drugs prescribed by a doctor and that does not necessary imply addiction. Dependence per se is not addiction. One can even be severely addicted without being proportionately dependent.

Addiction is a relapsing illness spanning a long period of time. Withdrawal is temporary and typically lasts from a few days to weeks. Most people, after coming out of withdrawal with or without treatment, would pick up their normal life from where they had left it. They may never take that drug or more significantly, take it occasionally without getting addicted.

The central feature of addiction is not withdrawal but an intense desire to take the drug, an overpowering urge called 'craving' in addiction parlance. Craving is worse when a person is exposed to cues in his environment, which remind him of the drug. These cues could include the sight of a harmless silver foil or a liquor shop, being in the presence of someone who is smoking or even just looking at an ash tray.

While tobacco addiction is one of the most intractable drug addictions and certainly the most damaging to the human body, quitting smoking leads to minimal or no withdrawal; it is the *intense craving,* which makes smoking difficult to stop as anybody who has tried to give up the habit would know. With cannabis, meth and LSD too, withdrawal is mild or non-existent, but it is the compelling craving, which makes addiction to these drugs tenacious.

~

Availability and social sanction are crucial factors in determining who and how many will start using a drug. A drug has to be available for people to take it. For example, in many Islamic countries, alcohol is not just frowned upon, but stringently prohibited. There are no liquor shops or bars and it is not served in restaurants. Selling alcohol invites strict punishment like lashes and long prison sentences.

In such countries, the proportion of people who drink and even more importantly, the proportion of people who start drinking young, is much smaller because getting hold of liquor is difficult. That much is a given advantage of prohibition. However, despite the hurdles some people would find the drug, but that number would be small. Even then, out of that small number who drink, the proportion or percentage of people who later become alcoholic would approximately be the same as in another country where there is no prohibition. Of course, both the absolute numbers of people who drink and that of people who are addicted to alcohol would be much smaller in an Islamic country than in other countries.

But this is not to say that very few people drinking alcohol and even fewer people becoming alcoholics means that the same holds true for people using and getting addicted to other drugs, which are not prohibited or looked down upon as much, such as tobacco and opium. Let us take the example of Pakistan, India's next-door neighbour and an Islamic country.

According to a report by UNODC titled 'Drug Use in Pakistan 2013', 6.7 million Pakistanis use drugs. A staggering 4.25 million are thought to be drug dependent. According to another report published in 2014 in the Asia-Pacific magazine *Diplomat*, in the country's north-western province of Khyber Pakhtunkhwa, an estimated 11% of residents use illicit substances–primarily heroin. The report says, 'Peshawar, the provincial capital of Khyber Pakhtunkhwa, is a city rife with homeless addicts and dirty needles.' Pakistan's KPK province has a long porous border with Afghanistan and opium is grown abundantly on both sides of the border. But there are very few alcoholics there.

According to the National Survey conducted in India in 2019, 0.74% of all Indians are dependent on drugs other than alcohol. According to the UNODC report mentioned above, in Pakistan, 2.4% of all Pakistanis are dependent on drugs.

The population of Pakistan is one-seventh of that of India. But Pakistan has half as many persons who inject heroin, proportionately three-and-a-half times more than India. On the other hand, while only 1.2% of the people in Pakistan had a drink in the previous year, 14.6% of Indians did. These figures tell us that while prohibition and unavailability of some intoxicants do lead to smaller numbers of people taking them and consequently smaller numbers of people getting addicted to them, it does not decrease the quantum of overall addiction in the community. In fact, people resort to other drugs which may be even more dangerous than the ones prohibited.

Addiction is thus like a large, soft balloon; if you press it at one point, it swells up elsewhere. The total quantum of addiction in any country remains the same. If you prohibit one drug people become addicted to another drug (or behaviour).

While countries do get to choose their intoxicants, they do not get to decrease the total quantum of addiction.

~

Virtually all drugs of addiction have common effects on a *single* pathway deep within the brain. This pathway, called the reward system, extends from the midbrain to the forebrain, with in turn connects to areas such as the limbic system and the orbitofrontal cortex. Activation of this reward system is what keeps drug users taking drugs. The reward is the feeling of pleasure often described as a 'high'. All addictive substances and addictive behaviours affect this circuit. This brain circuit also happens to be the same part of the brain, which is responsible for normal motivation and the desire for a reward.

Normally, to activate the reward system, a person involves himself in hard work or the pursuit of a hobby which brings pleasure, but that sustained diligence takes some time before it brings a reward.

Drugs (and certain behaviours) indulged in excess activate the reward system directly and instantaneously. These circuits provide a rush of positive feeling and feel-good chemicals to instantaneously 'reward' drug use. Thus, drugs provide a shortcut to pleasure by causing an intense activation of the reward system, which indirectly leads to neglect of work, family and friends because the reward can now be obtained through a shorter, much easier route. One does not have to 'work' for it.

However, these short cuts to pleasure are subject to the law of diminishing returns. Repeated intake of pleasure-giving drugs produces certain lasting changes in the reward system of the brain. Higher and higher doses are now required over time to produce less and less pleasure. Thus, drug use over time alters the brain in such a manner that less pleasure is elicited by not just by the same amount of the drug as before but also by the same amount of other pleasurable activities like sex, eating a favourite dessert or spending quality time with family. This is because the part of the brain responsible for the experience of pleasure is the same for the two seemingly very diverse sets of activities. As a result of the repetitive intake of the drug, the pleasure-giving part of the brain becomes blunted in its response to *all pleasurable activities* not just drug intake.

The pre-frontal cortex is the anterior-most part of the brain located just behind the forehead and above the eyeballs. Among many functions, including the finer traits of our personality like empathy and sensitivity, it is also responsible for the perception of stress, discretion, judgement and self-control. The pre-frontal cortex also undergoes long-term changes during addiction. This contributes to two things, which are the hallmark of addiction. One is impaired self-control and lack of inhibition in general, contributing to the person getting tempted too easily and making it difficult for him to stay away from the intoxicant. The other is the heightened perception of stress and decreased adaptation to it. The perceived stress can be current or even from incidents in the remote past like during childhood. This is how childhood deprivations, trauma and abuse contribute to increased chances of developing addictions. To make matters worse, due to these changes in the pre-frontal cortex, even routine stress is now perceived as catastrophic and unmanageable whether the stressful events are ongoing or they happened a long time ago.

Prolonged drug use causes pervasive changes in the brain that persist long after the individual stops taking the drug. Significant effects of chronic use have been identified for many drugs at all levels—at the level of molecules, brain cells and in the physical structure of specific parts of the brain. The *addicted brain thus is different from the non-addicted brain* along many parameters, and this is being proven by PET scans and other imaging tests of brain structure and functions. These changes are long lasting. Some of these are peculiar to specific drugs, whereas most are common to all drugs.

In short, different categories of drugs like heroin, alcohol, meth and ganja produce very different experiences, but when taken repeatedly over a long time, changes are produced in the same areas of the brain no matter which drug is used. These are the areas concerned with reward, pleasure, motivation, discretion, judgement and managing stress. The commonality of effects on the brain suggests that whatever the drug being used, the mechanisms are common to all addictions. *Addiction is tied to changes in brain structure and brain function and this is what makes it, fundamentally, a brain disease.* These changes are not present in casual users of drugs. A metaphorical switch in the brain seems to be flicked as a result of a combination of prolonged drug use plus predisposition to addiction, both of which are necessary pre-requisites. To start with, drug use is a voluntary behaviour, but when that switch is flicked, the individual moves into the state of addiction marked by compulsive drug use to the exclusion of all other activities in life.

It is believed that these changes in the brain may leave those with addiction vulnerable to physical and environmental cues that they associate with substance use even after treatment. When it comes to addiction, the world of an average addict contains a large number of cues. Whichever way the person turns, in his own house or in his social milieu, there is an abundance of cues. The chair on which he used to sit and drink is a cue, an ashtray is a cue, his authoritative boss is a cue, walking past a wine shop is a cue...This is the rationale for the concept of rehab as a part of the treatment of addiction. In rehab, after active medical treatment is over, the person lives for some time in a place where people are supportive but emotionally neutral and the place has no environmental triggers. He is asked to give it time before venturing out into his earlier surroundings, which is replete with triggers and cues.

~

Once addiction is established, the day-to-day behaviour of an individual with addiction develops a cyclical pattern with each cycle divided into three phases, which overlap to some extent. The cycle keeps on repeating as if it has a life of its own:

1. Phase of *preoccupation and anticipation*. Preoccupation is a continuous stream of thoughts about the drug; about how to get it and whether there is enough of it around. Thoughts also revolve around drug paraphernalia such as foil, syringe, needle, soda, ice, salted peanuts, etc.

2. Phase of *binge intoxication*. This is the actual period of drug use, drinking, snorting, inhaling, smoking and injecting, alone or with others.

3. *Withdrawal and negative effects*. This is when the drug levels in the blood stream are ebbing and its effects waning. It is a stage of unpleasant symptoms, guilt and self-deprecation (typified by the morning after a binge of heavy drinking over a long weekend), but in a person with drug addiction, it may be more frequent. This cycle is followed by another and they gradually escalate into a spiral, which then takes on a life of its own. This is what people mean by the dramatic expression, 'drugs hijack the brain.'

This expression explains the immense pull drugs exert on a person with addiction and how he has no time or energy to devote to other tasks and to people in his life. There is an inversion of previous priorities and an utter helplessness in being able to correct things. But like all simplifications this expression too obliterates the nuances. Take the case of thousands of American soldiers returning from the Vietnam War in the 70s. They could and did rescue their so-called 'hijacked' brains from drugs after being addicted.

Or so it seemed.

Heroin has a well-earned notoriety for being a highly addictive drug. It is common knowledge that a large number of American soldiers fighting the Vietnam War during the late 60s and early 70s were regularly taking heroin. In addition, they also used barbiturates and amphetamines. Before being recruited into the army, only 1% of them had used drugs on a regular basis. The obvious causes were the brutal and dangerous conditions on the warfront in addition to their being away from home and being emotionally isolated. The War quickly lost its meaning for those fighting it in faraway jungles on the other side of the globe. The disenchantment was made worse by the massive anti-war protests which swept across the USA. When the soldiers read about them in the papers, what they were doing seemed even more of a futile endeavour.

In 1971 when US Representatives Robert Steele and Morgan Murphy returned from an official visit to Vietnam, they came with news that stunned the American public: 15% of the active soldiers were heroin addicts. Given President Richard Nixon's promises to both end the war in Vietnam and solve the rising domestic crime rate, this news was especially unsettling.

When the war was coming to an end, the US government made extensive arrangements to treat the large number of presumed soldier addicts who would be returning home.

To start with, the Nixon administration ordered the military to start testing the soldiers who were still in Vietnam for heroin intake. No one could board a flight back to the US until he had cleared a urine test. Those who failed were to go through an army-sponsored detoxification programme named Operation Golden Flow. Men whose urine tested drug positive before departure were to be held back and detoxified for five to seven days until they had at least two clean urine samples. Only then could they board a plane headed to the United States.

Given the extraordinary addictiveness of heroin, nobody had high expectations about the long-term outcome of the intervention and most of the soldiers were expected to relapse. However, to everyone's surprise, Operation Golden Flow succeeded. When the word of the new dictate had spread, most soldiers stopped using narcotics. Almost all the soldiers who were detained passed the test on their second try if not the first.

Once they were back home, heroin lost its attraction. Heroin may have helped them endure a war's alternating spells of boredom and existential fears, but back in America, civilian life took precedence. Moreover, the sordid drug culture in the US, the prohibitive price of heroin and apprehensions of arrest discouraged them. Lee Robins, the Washington University sociologist who evaluated the testing programme, found that just 5% of the men who became addicted in Vietnam relapsed within ten months after return, and 12% relapsed briefly within three years.

Operation Gold Flow is an unprecedented success in the history of recovery programmes. Since it was the environment which had turned the tables, alteration in the environment of a person with addiction went on to become a standard component in the approach to treatment of addiction for many behavioural scientists after this.

Robins wrote, 'This surprising rate of recovery even when re-exposed to narcotic drugs ran counter to the conventional wisdom that heroin is a drug which causes addicts to suffer intolerable craving that rapidly leads to re-addiction if re-exposed to the drug.' Scholars hailed the results as 'revolutionary' and 'path-breaking'. The fact that addicts could quit heroin and remain drug-free also overturned the belief that 'once an addict, always an addict.' The remission rate was 95%, unheard of among narcotic addicts treated in the US or elsewhere. It also clearly showed that emotional isolation, powerlessness and stress are the conditions that promote addiction and when reversed, are sure to lead to recovery.

Project Golden Flow and the scientific studies based on it have been used as a strong argument by sociologists and psychologists to stress on two factors as crucial in addiction:

1. Environmental reasons are vital in the development, sustenance and termination of addiction.

2. Choice is important in getting people out of addiction. Once the soldiers knew they would not be able to board the plane to go back home to their families in the US till they gave up addiction, they chose to snap out of it and managed to stay out of it as well.

The Vietnam study of returning army men seems to complement the Rat Park study by the Canadian psychologist Bruce Alexander in which experimental rats when given a choice, preferred a socially stimulating environment to taking cocaine even after having experienced the latter's pleasurable effects. These two studies have been widely used by psychologists and sociologists to bring home the importance of social and environmental factors in the causation of drug addiction and contest the currently predominant medical model according to which addiction is a chronic remitting and relapsing disease like bronchial asthma, arthritis, hypertension and diabetes.

The logic of these psychologists and sociologists goes like this:

If addiction is a disease, you cannot get yourself out of it whenever you want like the American soldiers who fought in the Vietnam War apparently did when faced with the choice to give up addiction or stay behind in Vietnam. However, in response, the proponents of the biological causation of addiction or the medical model point out that while the cohort of Vietnam War returnees did show stunning rates of recovery, this was and remains so far, the only study of its kind. These results have not been replicated even once in the last fifty years in the hundreds of studies conducted since then.

It is argued that heroin use during the Vietnam War

happened under exceptionally abysmal and stressful conditions. The soldiers were exposed to a vicious war, which was considered meaningless by Americans back home. It was being fought in a location where heroin was cheap and easily available. Some of the soldiers took it regularly and since heroin is a strong drug and the one available in Vietnam was of particularly good quality, a good number of them became *dependent* in the sense that when they did not take it, they experienced classic withdrawal symptoms giving the impression that they were addicted. But they were just physiologically dependent on it without being addicted in the true sense like the thousands of patients of heroin addiction, who were being treated in various addiction clinics across the US.

Probably, the best comparison that can be drawn is to situational homosexual behaviour seen in boys' camps in remote locations where a large number of young men live in close proximity and heterosexual behaviour is not an option. Since homosexual activity is never the preferred sexual behaviour, once the camp ends and people go back home, homosexual behaviour 'disappears'. This does not by any stretch of the imagination mean that sexual orientation can be called a matter of picking an option or that it can be mastered by will power and choice or that it can be changed using a tough approach.

One can also point out that the American soldiers who fought in Vietnam were not a strictly representative sample of the general population of the United States or anywhere else. They had passed tough medical examinations, gone through rigorous training and successfully endured one of the toughest wars in history in one of the most inhospitable terrains that the US army had ever been exposed to. Results from such a niche population selected for their above average physical and psychological constitution cannot be applicable to the general population.

The current model of addiction thus remains that of a primary, chronic disease characterized by impaired control over the use of drugs with environmental factors perpetuating and worsening the disease. Like other chronic diseases, it can be progressive, relapsing and even fatal. To understand addictions, we have to look beyond drugs, howsoever strong they may be. As Lance Dodes, a psychiatrist at the Harvard Medical School Division of Addictions rightly pointed out, 'Addiction is a human problem that resides in people, not in the drug or in the drug's capacity to produce physical effects.'

CHAPTER 9

Behavioural Addictions: Addictions Without Drugs

The thing that hit me other than the freezing air on entering the air-conditioned train coach that summer morning was the sight of several men clad in spotless white clothes and turbans crowding the aisle. I was heading home from Delhi by the morning Shatabdi Express after attending a weekend seminar in the capital city. The men in white had come to see off an old man wearing holy robes, who reclined in his seat with several garlands around his neck and strings of beads on his wrists. The men made way for me grudgingly which made me feel so much like an interloper that I checked my ticket to make sure I was in the right coach. My seat was two rows behind that of the godman.

Suddenly, there was a commotion at the entrance and a young woman dressed in a white sari and a rather tastefully designed diamond necklace pushed past the men crowding the aisles, and dropped at the feet of the holy man. Clutching the sacred feet, she pleaded that she had become so used to seeing her god for six blissful months that her soul would wither away without a *darshan* (sighting) every morning. She begged him to stay or to take her along with him. Tears rolling down her pretty face which was now contorted in agony, she wailed nonstop. Her cries attracted the train superintendent's attention. He peeped in to see if everything was alright. He must have seen similar scenes before since he backed away coolly after a couple of minutes.

The godman, however, kept staring vacantly into the distance as if nothing unusual was happening. His followers too looked unmoved. Eventually, he did make some weak gestures at his followers to take the woman away. Just then, another young man in white, breathless from running, entered the coach. With folded hands, he apologized to the godman for his wife's behaviour. He said that she had extracted the car keys from under his pillow while he was sleeping and driven away. The guru nodded his pardon, and the woman, kicking and wailing, was carried out of the coach by the husband and some volunteers.

As the engine gave a loud honk, the men wearing sparkling white kurta pyjamas and exorbitantly expensive watches bowed deferentially before the holy man and left. The train glided out of the station and except for Guruji's entourage fussing over his honey, milk and other paraphernalia, normalcy was restored. As is one's wont on return journeys from Delhi, I went over my notes as the train chugged along. The previous day's seminar on 'Internet Addiction' had been the reason for my trip. A discussant had objected saying that the whole concept seemed to be hype, a case of overkill, and in her words, 'yet another attempt by medical professionals to pathologize normal behaviour, in this case, humankind's honest attempts to match the rapid pace of technology.'

The main speaker, however, had replied fairly convincingly that people who wake up thrice a night to check their WhatsApp messages, keep an eye on their Facebook page while having sex and suffer intense craving if the Wi-Fi stops working, certainly need help. He went on to display some slides to show that the same areas of the brain involved in persons addicted to drugs like heroin were involved here as well.

When I met my friend and fellow psychiatrist Bobby the following Saturday evening, I talked about the seminar to him. He, in turn, told me about the couple he had seen the previous week who runs a successful courier company and has a correctly self-diagnosed stock market addiction. Whatever they earned from their business, and it was plenty, they blew it promptly on stocks. The two spent their nights studying the behaviour patterns of securities, following stock experts on the internet, calculating the positions of the stars and buying securities online at the exact auspicious moment even if that happened to be 2 a.m. Nothing worked, of course. But that did not stop them. They slept little, neglected their children and had no time or energy to get them to school in time. Bills had been mounting and banks were breathing down their necks. Bobby being a good professional did not tell me their names, nor did I ask. Ours is a small city and I practically know everyone who lives here.

I moved on to the topic of the train journey where everybody in the coach except me was dressed in white and wore flashy watches. I described the young woman's condition to Bobby.

With an amused twinkle in his eyes, Bobby asked. 'So, you think she too was an addict?'

'Why not? She behaved like one.'

'And that eighty-year-old godman with a zillion followers, a peddler?'

'Well, he behaved like one.'

'Maybe,' he agreed tentatively but had a question. 'What about the crowd of men in white who had come to see him off. They behaved normally, didn't they?'

'Maybe they were all casual users and she was the only one with an addiction.'

'Touché,' Bobby conceded.

Bobby is a fair man indeed!

~

To understand addiction well, one must look at the seemingly radical but well-proven fact that drugs are not a sine-qua-non for addiction; that addiction can occur without drugs. Out of the two words, 'drug' and 'addiction', the crucial word is addiction, not the drug. Also, drug addiction is just one among many forms of addiction.

The concept of 'behavioural addiction' provides the most important bridge yet in understanding the true nature of addiction. Behavioural addiction is not just a loose and lackadaisical bandying of terms like workaholic or sex addict, to describe someone whom we do not like. Behavioural addictions are as disabling, destructive and disempowering as drug addictions and as much of an illness. In August 2011, the American Society of Addiction Medicine (ASAM) issued a public statement giving a new definition of addiction. It said,

'Addiction is a primary, chronic disease of brain involving reward, motivation, memory and related circuitry.' Note that there is no reference to any drug or substance in the definition. This was the first time the ASAM adopted the official position that addiction was not solely drug addiction, and that 'addiction' can also be a reference to excessive 'behaviours' that are rewarding.

This definition basically reiterated that the structure and functions of brain circuits of persons with addiction to a drug *or* to a behaviour, differ from the structure and function of the brain circuits of persons who do not have any addiction. And that while the brain of a person with addiction is different from that of a person without addiction, the brain of a person with drug addiction is similar to that of a person with behavioural addictions.

Eating, sexual behaviour and gambling behaviour among others can be associated with the 'pathological pursuit of rewards' described in this new definition of addiction. All of us have the normal reward circuitry in our brains that makes food and sex pleasurable and rewarding. It is essential for survival that everybody finds food interesting. If people did not find sex (essential for the propagation of the species) pleasurable, they would not bother to have sex.

In a normal brain, these rewards have feedback mechanisms for satiety which signals 'enough' at a certain point. In someone with addiction, the circuitry becomes dysfunctional and the message to the individual becomes 'more', which leads to a compulsive pursuit of rewards through drugs, eating, sex or other behaviours like gambling and video gaming. Since the seat of addiction in the brain is common to drug and behavioural addiction, an individual who has drug addiction is also vulnerable to behavioural addiction and vice versa because the same parts of the brain are involved.

Thus, behavioural addiction involves a compulsion to engage in a rewarding behaviour despite negative consequences to the person's physical, mental, social or financial well-being. In behavioural addictions too exactly the same cycles of pleasure-anticipation, binge-intoxication and stress-withdrawal occur repeatedly, triggering a spiral of addiction behaviour. Behavioural addictions are increasingly recognized as treatable along the same lines as drug addiction. The excessive behaviours which have so far been identified as being addictive include gambling, eating, sexual intercourse, use of pornography, playing video games, excessive exercise, shopping, cosmetic surgery and excessive tanning.

We know that out of the many people who drink or take weed only a small proportion are alcoholics or addicted to weed. Similarly, out of the large number of people who gamble or play video games, only a very small minority are addicted to these behaviours. But the small number who are, are addicted just like a heroin addict, showing all the typical qualities of addiction like intense preoccupation, craving and excessive indulgence which leads them to ignore all aspects of their lives. Work and family time are side-lined and addiction proceeds relentlessly at the cost of the individual's health, relationships and finances. That particular behaviour acquires *salience*, a red beacon burning dangerously bright like the compelling attraction Odysseus felt for the Sirens in Homer's classic.

Out of the behavioural addictions, gambling addiction and gaming addiction have already been categorized as addictive disorders in the World Health Organization's 2018 International Classification of Diseases (ICD). Gambling addiction is also featured in the DSM-5, the latest list of diseases used in the US and Canada. If somebody is diagnosed as having a gambling addiction or a gaming addiction, he can go to a hospital and get treated for it just like a person with heroin addiction. Some insurance companies and employers in many countries even reimburse the expenses and others are on their way to.

However, it is vital to recognise the fact that all the people who gamble are not suffering from addiction disorder, in fact, only a small proportion are, just as everybody who drinks is not an alcoholic, only a minority are. According to the DSM-5, the following criteria have to be fulfilled before someone can be diagnosed as having gambling addiction:

Persistent and recurrent problematic gambling behaviour

leading to clinically significant impairment or distress, as indicated by the individual exhibiting four or more of the following in the previous twelve-month period:

1) Needs to gamble with increasing amounts of money in order to achieve the desired excitement.

2) Is restless or irritable when attempting to cut down or stop gambling.

3) Has made repeated unsuccessful efforts to control, cut back or stop gambling.

4) Is often preoccupied with gambling (persistent thoughts of reliving past gambling experiences, handicapping or planning the next venture, thinking of ways to get money with which to gamble).

5) Often gambles when feeling distressed.

6) Often goes back to gamble after losing money to get even (i.e., 'chasing' one's losses).

7) Lies to conceal the extent of involvement with gambling.

8) Has jeopardized or lost a significant relationship, job, or educational or career opportunity because of gambling.

9) Relies on others to provide money to fix desperate financial situations caused by gambling.

Interestingly, in each of the above nine points, if the word 'gambling' is substituted by 'heroin intake', nobody will have the slightest difficulty in understanding that we are talking of a fairly advanced case of heroin addiction.

In 2018, ignoring the protests from the rich and powerful gaming industry, the WHO recognized gaming addiction as a disease and included it in its classification of diseases. Again, most people who enjoy video gaming are not gaming addicts. For gaming disorder to be diagnosed the following criteria are necessary according to the WHO:

A pattern of persistent or recurrent gaming behaviour

(digital gaming or video gaming), which may be online or offline, manifested by:

1. Impaired control over gaming e.g., onset, frequency, intensity, duration, termination, context, often more than one of these.

2. Increasing priority given to gaming to the extent that gaming takes precedence over all other life interests and daily activities (like studies, examinations, work, relationships, etc.) and

3. Continuation or escalation of gaming despite the occurrence of negative consequences (like failing in exams, problems at work, marital problems). The behaviour pattern is of sufficient severity to result in significant impairment in personal, family, social, educational, occupational or other important areas of functioning.

(The examples in parentheses under 2 and 3 have been added by me.)

In India, many gaming apps are available and are being advertised through slick commercials featuring popular movie actors. Ironically, these commercials come with the warning that gaming can lead to addiction and can drain your financial resources. Psychiatrists in the country are already treating gaming addicts in their clinics and if the trend continues it may become a major mental health problem of our time. To make the issue more complex, since one can also bet on the outcomes of games, this addiction in some youngsters leads to a combination of gaming and gambling addictions.

After schools and colleges closed down in March 2020 because of the Covid-19 pandemic, there was an increase in the incidence of gaming addiction in India. One startling incident comes to mind—India.com on July 5, 2020 reported the case of a fifteen-year-old boy from Mohali, Punjab who spent two lakh rupees on Player Unknown's Battlegrounds (PUBG), which he had transferred out of his grandfather's pension account.

While other behavioural addictions are not given a separate code each by the WHO or the DSM, these can be categorized as 'other specified disorders due to addictive behaviours' if these behavioural addictions fulfil the rest of the criteria described in the case of gambling addiction or gaming addiction. The theoretical and practical significance of behavioural addictions finding a listing in the WHO's ICD or North America's DSM is immense.

Decades of research conducted by leading universities and hospitals across the world and then published in peer-reviewed medical journals of repute followed by months of rigorous debates and discussions within the WHO precede the listing of a new condition as a disease. This is because the implications of such a listing are of great significance. The fact that health insurance companies sooner or later will have to reimburse the expenses incurred in treating these diseases is one among them. While gambling and gaming addictions are already accorded the status of medical illnesses by the WHO, certain other behaviours like eating, sex, shopping and exercise are being researched for their potential for being addictive in a small minority of persons although these happen to be behaviours essential for survival and normal living.

It is important to note that whether it is gambling or eating or sex, the thinking about their compulsive and damaging versions being addictions did not happen overnight as a sudden fad. Although pathological gambling was designated an addiction only in 2013, the medical journal, *Journal of Gambling Behaviour* was started way back in 1985.

The term 'food addiction' has been studied for its commonalities to substance and behavioural addictions. The only controversy is whether what we have here is more of a substance addiction than behaviour addiction, the substance being high-fat, high-sugar and high-salt foods. Foods which are not high in fat, sugar or salt do not lead to binge eating or food addiction. Scientists at Yale University, in fact, have devised a Food Addiction Scale. This twenty-five-item self-report measurement has been developed to identify those who are most likely to have food addiction. A food addiction symptom count (e.g., tolerance, withdrawal and loss of control) can be calculated, which is similar to the criteria for drug addiction. Some excerpts from the self-rating Yale Food Addiction Scale are listed below to illustrate similarities with other addictions:

*I find myself continuing to consume certain foods even though I am no longer hungry.

*I eat to the point where I feel physically ill.

*I spend a lot of time feeling sluggish or fatigued from overeating.

*There have been times when I consumed certain foods so often or in such large quantities that *I started to eat food instead of working, spending time with my family or friends, or engaging in other important activities or recreational activities I enjoy.*

*I have had *withdrawal symptoms* such as agitation, anxiety, or other physical symptoms when I cut down or stopped eating certain foods.

*I experience significant problems in my ability to function effectively (daily routine, job/school, social activities, family activities, health) because of food and eating.

*My food consumption has caused significant psychological or physical problems

*Over time, I have found that *I need to eat more and more to feel the same degree of pleasure.*

Sociologists have pointed to the longstanding relationship

between addictions and commerce. Historically, without labourers and other workers with addiction, some of whom were paid in kind for producing the very substance to which they were addicted, the markets in tobacco, caffeine, opium, cannabis, and coca products may not have come into being. In the light of food being an addiction, we can add the fast-food market to the list. Low-wage-earning fast-food workers who toil away in shifts often take advantage of readily available, cheap fast-food saturated with fat and salt, because it suits their schedules and their incomes and is economical for their employers too.

The term 'sex addiction' has been used even more commonly than 'food addiction'. It is also called compulsive sexual behaviour (CSB) or hypersexuality and is recognized by repetitive and intense preoccupations with sexual fantasies, urges and behaviours that are distressing to the individual and result in functional impairment. Individuals with CSB often know their sexual behaviour to be excessive but are unable to control it. CSB can involve fantasies and urges in addition to or in place of the actual behaviour but it must cause significant distress to the person before it can be called an addiction. It must also cause interference in daily life to qualify as a disorder. The so-called 'porn addiction' is a variety of sex addiction.

Another upcoming behavioural addiction is addiction to excessive exercise and extreme sports. Despite risk of severe physical injury or death, participation in extreme sports such as skydiving, downhill skiing and rock climbing continues to grow. Participating athletes are often referred to as 'adrenaline junkies'. Using a twenty-four-item addiction questionnaire with dimensions including preoccupation, self-medication and the occurrence of physical injuries, it was found that addiction was strongly related to skydivers' length of exposure to the extreme sport. Extreme sports athletes commonly describe a 'rush' or 'high' when taking part in their sport and liken these experiences to those of drug intake. Skydivers have described their sport as being 'like an addiction,' stating that they 'can't get enough,' and some say that their relationships suffer as a result.

Behavioural addictions being at par with drug addictions, involving the same specific brain changes, is a game changer in understanding the nature of addiction because it frees us from the shackles of viewing only drugs as the key to addiction. We now know that *drugs are neither sufficient nor necessary causes of addiction*. With that, the focus shifts to the personality of the individual and his environment. The individual is no longer an inert human who happens to take drugs a few times and ends up with his brain being hijacked by drugs as the popular narrative goes. This narrative is an overdramatic simplification as well as misleading. And it is wrong science too. It mistakenly deflects all the societal resources into slaying the demon, which is a particular set of drugs, by trying to cut off their supply using the harsh strictures of the criminal justice system. Here, the hope is that when there are no drugs, there will be no addictions. The long-drawn War on Drugs is as good as lost. Even if we had slain that demon and won that war and even if the world had been rid of all intoxicating drugs, we would still have addictions in the form of behavioural addictions, which can be as devastating as drug addictions.

Behavioural addictions are likely to change the commonly perceived profile of a person with addiction. A perfectly well-dressed man or woman in a shopping mall craving 'retail therapy', a woman waiting for her fifth cosmetic surgery in a swanky clinic, a middle-aged man regularly using his office computer to watch porn thus risking his job, a group of young businessmen from a mid-sized city waiting to board a flight to Kathmandu for their next gambling trip to casinos from where some of them will come back devastated, but will go back again—any of them could be suffering from a behavioural addiction. In other words, this brings the addictions home for the upper middle class. It is no longer something that 'others' suffer from. Any of us could be one of 'them'.

As renowned Canadian addiction specialist and author Gabor Maté notes, 'In our materialistic society, with our attachment to ego gratification, few of us escape the lure of addictive behaviours. Only our blindness and self-flattery stand in the way of seeing that the severely addicted are people who have suffered more than the rest of us but who share a profound commonality with the majority of "respectable citizens"'.

Maté goes on to say in his now canonical book, *In the Realm of Hungry Ghosts: Close Encounters with Addiction,* 'No society can understand itself without looking at its shadow side. I believe there is one addiction process, whether it is manifested in the lethal substance dependencies of my downtown East Side patients; the frantic self-soothing of overeaters or shopaholics; the obsessions of gamblers, sexaholics and compulsive Internet users; or the socially acceptable and even admired behaviours of the workaholic.'

~

I had an interesting client in the late '70s—a colleague from the medical field—when I was working at my first job at the Christian Medical College in Ludhiana. When he called to fix up his appointment, he had said he wanted my opinion about whether or not he needed to stop drinking, which was an unusual reason for a psychiatric consultation. So, I looked forward to meeting him with some degree of curiosity. He was a much sought-after general physician of the city. Dr Kohli, (let me call him that), was seventy years old and had been drinking two large pegs of whiskey every day for the last fifty years. 'Every day, 120 ml,' he emphasised. 'For *fifty* years.'

He didn't skip his drink on Hindu religious festivals or fasts nor on Tuesdays and Thursdays. Many people who drink regularly abstain for religious reasons during these times. Tuesdays and Thursdays are given a miss, again for religious reasons. Some wait to get together with their buddies to drink but that did not apply to Dr Kohli since he drank alone at home.

Dr Kohli on an average saw fifty patients in a day, a hundred during the two months of dengue season. He remembered their names and the names of their family members most of whom were also his patients. He made four to five home visits, lanced abscesses, dressed wounds, was never late for work, worked Sunday mornings too, but did not go on home visits at night. Night visits are a very important part of a GP's work because families depend upon their GP for dealing with health emergencies which may crop up at night.

'Do you have withdrawal or craving if you do not drink?' I asked him, naively, as it turned out.

'I wouldn't know, that has never happened,' he replied in a matter-of-fact manner.

He spent the evenings with his family members none of whom had a problem with his drinking. He watched TV with them every evening and that is when he had his drink. In fact, his wife or his daughter-in-law would pick up his whiskey when they went to buy groceries. He only had two drinks, never more, not even at weddings. He woke up at five daily and never missed his morning walk. And all his tests—including liver function tests—came back normal.

Whenever he travelled for conferences which he was fond

of attending, he travelled light with one bag which contained some clothes, toiletries, a bottle of whiskey (those were pre-9/11 days, bottles were allowed) and his cocktail snacks. He said flights often got delayed, room service in hotels was painfully slow and his brand of Scotch was difficult to get when he was travelling. He stuck to two drinks, which he measured using a peg measure he carried in his bag. He calculated his peg with the same methodical attitude with which he prepared cough mixtures for his patients and wrote his prescriptions.

I asked him if he thought about alcohol when he was working.

'I do,' he said candidly. 'I have never taken a sip at work, I cannot even think of doing that, but after five, most of my thoughts are about drinking—the paraphernalia—bottle, soda, ice, scrambled eggs, etc.'

In the end, he asked me, 'So, do you think I am an alcoholic? Should I give up?'

I honestly told him those were two different questions. Whether to give up or not in his case was a question of personal choice because only he could decide if he was getting more from alcohol than he was giving it—he was a doctor himself. About being an alcoholic or not, I said he was a stable alcoholic but that label, at his age and functional level, was irrelevant.

'Why do you think I am an alcoholic or could be one?' he asked.

'Because you do not have a "take it or leave it" attitude towards alcohol. You do not go on night visits because of your drinking and night visits are important because you are a GP and your patients cannot depend on you in case of emergencies. Also, because you have a compulsion for and a preoccupation with alcohol. There is anticipation and insecurity, you do not go anywhere without your bottle, the cocktail snacks and the peg measure. You think a lot about drinking even when you are not drinking? Your mind space is cluttered with thoughts about alcohol.'

There was a longish pause.

Finally, he said something totally unexpected, 'By the criterion of mind space and how much of it one allocates to alcohol, I think our respected Prime Minister although a simple and selfless man, is a bigger alcoholic than me.'

This was the late 70s and newspapers frequently carried articles on the anti-alcohol rhetoric of the then Prime Minister.

Dr Kohli added, 'All the man seems to think about during his waking and sleeping hours is alcohol and how immoral it is and how the country should ban it. Against the sane advice of his cabinet ministers, he has written to all states in the country to ban alcohol within four years. Wherever he goes he carries that message like a missionary. I think there is nothing else on his mind except alcohol. According to your criterion of mind space, he is an alcoholic since he is fanatic about it.'

He went on to share a medical analogy like a true GP. 'Could I be a pre-alcoholic, you know, like a pre-diabetic, like people who go through life with borderline glucose levels but never becoming a frank diabetic?'

I left him with that relatively comfortable thought.

Although I did not meet Dr Kohli again in person, I heard that he carried on with his two large pegs every day (sharp at 7.30 p.m.) till he was seventy-nine when he died in a car crash, with someone else driving. But through his kooky comparison, he did leave me with the insight that figuratively speaking, one can be a teetotaller and an alcoholic at the same time.

Several years later, I was at an Alcoholics Anonymous (AA) meeting, curious to know more about them. AA, founded in 1935, is an international organization which has done more good for persons with alcohol addiction than any other social organization. It is run by former alcoholics. A senior member who ran the branch introduced himself like this, 'I am Mr XYZ. I am an alcoholic.' I knew that the man had not touched alcohol for twenty years. But that is the way all AA members introduce themselves in their internal meetings. At the heart of the matter was the humility to accept that staying away from alcohol after having been an alcoholic takes effort and eternal vigilance. It a time-consuming job for anybody and a full-time job for those who run such an organization. For them it is a cause, not just a hobby.

Mind space for and fanaticism towards the cause are essential. Here, the cause is anti-alcohol, but alcohol is still in the equation. Of course, the cause here is something good for society. Second, while using a drug or alcohol may or may not be temporary, addiction is not. It is permanent, and relapses do happen.

The comparison of addiction to fanaticism may seem an overreach but it is easy to understand if we can, in our minds, manage to divest the concept of addiction of any moral overtones and value judgement. Thus, perceived from a morally neutral and purely scientific perspective, fanaticism of any kind is an 'addiction' too. An addiction which can be good for society like that of an ardent social reformer whose thoughts are consumed by the cause, often at the cost of his own health and to the exclusion of the welfare of his own near and dear ones. Many fanatics like these have changed the world for the better.

Being a believer in a cause is not necessarily being a fanatic like playing video games does not necessarily mean a gaming addiction and smoking weed is not necessarily a cannabis addiction. The person can take it or leave it depending upon other exigencies.

Fanaticism is a belief or behaviour involving uncritical zeal and an obsessive enthusiasm which brooks no reasoning or opposition. The content of the belief is not important, the form is. And the opposite of the religious fanatic is not the fanatical atheist. They are the same. The opposite of a religious fanatic is a gentle religious person or a gentle atheist. Both can be persuaded to be tolerant of the other's point of view while the religious fanatic and the fanatical atheist cannot be.

Fanatics to any cause cannot be moderately good or moderately bad for society. They are either very good like an ardent social reformer who changes the world for the better or very bad like a member of an extremist organization donning a suicide jacket. Interestingly, the same mechanism works to produce two diametrically opposite results.

CHAPTER 10

Why Do Some People Get Addicted and Others Do Not?

'Two identical seeds cultivated under opposing conditions would yield two different plants.'

—Gabor Maté, addiction expert and author

Addictions are a group of complex illnesses in which both genetic as well as environmental causes play their part. These diseases have a chronic and relapsing course with remissions lasting from days to years. Addictions typically appear as the uncontrolled and repetitive use of a drug or an activity, with outcomes harmful to the individual and those around him. Addictions demand exclusive rights to a person's time, effort and mind space and because of this overdemanding nature of the phenomena, addictions destroy work, family life and social relationships. Although consumption of addictive agents and involvement in addictive behaviours are voluntary, they sooner or later lead to volitional control being compromised because of the compulsive nature of addictions.

This chapter takes up a frequently asked question: to what extent are the processes involved in the initiation and maintenance of addiction influenced by genetics and to what extent by the environment?

In general, there are three types of genetic evidence which can tell us whether an illness is hereditary or not. These are:

1. Family Studies: If the occurrence of an illness is higher in the first-degree relatives (parents, siblings, children) of a person suffering from an illness as compared to the second-degree relatives (cousins, uncles, aunts, nephews, nieces), who in turn have higher rates as compared to the general population, it is strongly indicative that heredity has a role to play. However, close family members also share the same environment and so family studies alone may not be enough to prove that heredity is responsible for addictions any more than shared environment.

For example, if the parents drink, chances are high that bottles of whiskey or vodka may be lying around the house and be easily available to an adolescent. Chances are also high for the parents to be more tolerant of their child taking a sip once in a while than in a family where everybody is a teetotaller. So, how do we know if the reason is the parents' genes or their permissive attitude?

2. Adoption Studies: If children who are adopted soon after birth show a higher incidence of addictions when they grow up than the members of their adopted family and that incidence is more like the incidence in their biological family, it would mean that genetics plays a more important role in causing addictions than the environment. If the opposite is true, one would be correct in concluding that environmental factors are more important in causing addictions than genetic factors.

3. Twin Studies: Identical twins share genetic material which is the exact replica of each other, while non-identical twins, genetically speaking, are like regular siblings.

When both members of a pair of twins suffer from the

same illness, they are said to be concordant for that illness. If concordance rates for an illness in a series of identical twins are much higher than concordance rates in a series of non-identical twins, it is safe to assume that in the causation of that particular disease, genetic factors have a major role to play since the environment during early childhood is the same for both sets of twins.

In the case of addictions, family, adoption and twin studies all show that an individual's risk for addiction tends to be proportional to the degree of genetic relationship to a relative with addiction. Various genetic studies have shown that addictions have a moderate to high hereditability. A safe estimate would be that at least 50% of the burden of causation is shared by genetic factors and the rest by social and environmental factors such as the availability of drugs and stress.

A significant view on the shifting balance of genetic and environmental influences has been obtained from the developmental perspective. The Virginia Twin Study, in a series of publications, revealed that in early adolescence the initiation and use of nicotine, alcohol and cannabis are more strongly determined by familial and social factors like permissiveness and availability, but these gradually decline in importance during progression to young and middle adulthood, when the effects of genetic factors become the maximum.

As a broad rule, environmental and social factors like easy availability and social sanction are more important in initiating drug use at a young age and genetic factors play a more important part in determining who eventually becomes addicted and who does not. Simply put, if a drug is available during adolescence and parental controls lax, there are more chances of a young person using that drug but not all of them grow up to be addicted to those drugs. To a large extent, genetic factors determine who does and who does not.

The moderate to high heritability of addiction disorder is paradoxical because addictions initially depend on the availability of the addictive agent, and it is the individual's choice to use it or not. The availability of addictive agents is determined by the culture, social policy, religion, economic status and narco-trafficking, and it changes across time and place. Thus, the Twin Studies on addiction indicate that under particular societal scenarios, genes play a substantial role in causation of addictions. Like other complex diseases such as obesity, diabetes, cancer and coronary heart disease, addictions are strongly influenced by genetic background but also by lifestyle and individual choices.

However, what is inherited is a generic addiction trait, not the propensity to develop addiction to a specific drug or behaviour. In a genetically predisposed person, which drug or behaviour the person will get addicted to would depend totally upon access, permissiveness and the environment.

One summer, a couple of years back, a young man was brought by his parents and twin brother to my outpatients' clinic for treatment. It was a nuclear family unit, which was a part of an extended business family living in connected houses and involved in wool trade in the downtown part of the city. The patient was in his late twenties and had been using heroin for several years. He had been admitted multiple times to psychiatry and addiction treatment units at various city hospitals. Each of these admissions had resulted in remissions lasting a few weeks to a couple of months. Repeated questions by the resident psychiatrist about history of addictions in any other members of the family was met with indignant denials. This of course is possible, but here we had the patient's identical twin sitting right next to him, whom the family swore was totally unlike his brother—highly responsible, an ideal son and utterly devoid of any addiction.

I sensed that the young man (the ideal twin) had something in his mouth. As things unravelled, it came to light that he had been using tobacco for even longer than his twin brother had been snorting heroin. And a dentist's warning one year back after he discovered a suspicious patch of discoloured mucosa in his mouth had made no difference. Also, the father had been drinking half a bottle of whiskey every day for over fifteen years even after a diagnosis of inflammation of the oesophagus. None of them were considered by the family to be addicts since alcohol and tobacco were not thought to be addictions. Also, the patient's uncle, the father's brother, had left home at the age of twenty-five without telling anybody and was gone without a trace.

After fifteen years, a neighbour had spotted him in an ashram adjoining a temple in Haridwar with a group of ganja-smoking sadhus, whom he was living with. This indicated a mixed behaviour and drug addiction. When the family went to see him, he had met them cordially but refused to go back home saying that he was happy where he was. However, none of these three members of the family were considered to be suffering from an 'addiction' like the young man with heroin use. They were not even considered fit to be mentioned in the context of addictions even after being specifically asked about addiction in any other family member.

As for me, looking at the family afresh provided me with the possible genetic connection between the patient's heroin addiction, his twin brother's advanced nicotine addiction, his father's alcoholism and his uncle's behavioural and cannabis addiction.

Distress, Stress, Trauma and Addictions

That individuals seek drugs in pursuit of positive pleasure over and above their usual feeling state is only a part of the truth. Relief from a pre-existing distress is also a relative pleasure. Drugs relieve psychological distress as much as they relieve physical pain. In fact, relief from chronic distress is a far stronger and more common reason for resorting to drugs in persons who take drugs repeatedly (leading to addiction in some of them). Heroin and cocaine are both powerful painkillers, but they also numb emotional hurts and psychological distress borne out of past trauma. And that is why many people with clinically diagnosable depression, anxiety and PTSD take narcotic drugs as a way of self-medicating. The brain pathways which mediate physical pain are the same ones which mediate psychological distress as well. That is also the reason why persons who take drugs to relieve psychological pain find it more difficult to get rid of the habit because the underlying trauma, painful feelings and psychiatric conditions persist unless looked for and treated separately.

There are two life events which researchers have found to additionally increase the chances of an individual becoming addicted to drugs or ending up with behavioural addictions. A large number of studies show that both childhood sexual abuse and physical abuse are strongly co-related with the person developing addictive disorders later in life. In a Canadian study completed in 2016, data of 14,063 individuals reporting childhood sexual abuse was examined. Sexual abuse during childhood was found to be positively co-related with heavy drinking, hazardous drinking, use of marijuana and other illicit drugs. Child abuse, according to some, is as likely to cause drug addiction as obesity is to cause heart disease. One can only guess the shock and the sudden loss of credibility in a child's mind about an adult who was so far seen as a source of love, comfort and security. The study concluded that all societal measures which reduced child abuse would be expected to reduce addiction as well.

In another study on the relationship between child abuse and drug addiction conducted simultaneously in the USA and Australia, 84% respondents reported a history of childhood abuse or neglect. As Gabor Maté notes, 'Not all addictions are rooted in abuse or trauma, but I do believe they can all be traced to a painful experience. *A hurt is at the centre of all addictive behaviours.* The wound may not be as deep and the ache not as excruciating, and it may even be entirely hidden—but it's there...The drug restores to the addict the childhood vivacity she suppressed long ago.'

Early childhood trauma, apart from being a starkly traumatic event in itself, also determines how the person responds every time a stressful situation occurs in later life.

In short, depending upon the availability of a drug and other social factors like cultural sanction and peer pressure, a large number of people use drugs; however, a still larger number do not, ever. Only a small proportion of those who use drugs get addicted. They are predisposed to addiction because of either genetics or environmental factors like childhood neglect and abuse. In these persons, drugs produce structural and functional changes in certain specific parts of the brain which then take over and perpetuate the addiction spiral of anticipation, intoxication and its negative effects. This spiral in time gains a momentum of its own.

A distinguished psychiatrist colleague from Kolkata, Dr Bhaskar Mukherjee, summarised it succinctly in a piece of personal communication we shared:

*Addiction is a genetically transmitted trait of the brain which lasts for a person's whole life.

*Expression of that trait may be triggered by some adverse childhood experiences.

*Addiction is not confined to drugs. It is a tendency to pursue an activity which gives a person pleasure at the cost of the exclusion of everything else.

*Although a genetic trait, it is not normatively distributed like height or intelligence which everybody has, less or more. It is a non-normative trait—only some people have it and others do not have it at all.

CHAPTER 11

How Should a Country Manage Addictions?

Science has made remarkable progress in understanding addiction and its causes. Consequently, management of addiction has come a long way during last few decades and is no longer as frustrating for all concerned as it was before. Addiction is now understood and treated as an illness with a chronic remitting and relapsing course with long periods of remission. Like most chronic illnesses, it has a multi-factorial causation. There have been dramatic advances over the past three decades on the twin fronts of neurosciences and behavioural sciences, which have led to a radical change in our understanding of the nature of addiction. We already know the exact neural circuits through which every known drug of abuse acts. We know the common pathways in the brain that are used by almost all addictive drugs.

Science has also teased out and even cloned the receptors, the landing pads in the brain, which these drugs selectively latch on to after crossing the blood brain barrier. We are also well on our way to pinning down the major differences between the brains of addicted and non-addicted individuals. Scientists have also identified some common denominators of addiction regardless of the substance.

The three-pronged thrust of management of all addictions is:

i) Medication to first treat the withdrawal and then the longer-lasting craving.

ii) Psychotherapy and behaviour modification through stress handling and other psychological interventions like repairing broken relationships and working with families of the person with addiction.

iii) Social reintegration.

For opioid addiction, there are broadly two diametrically opposite types of medical treatments available:

A. *Abstinence oriented.* Here the patient needs to be admitted to a specialized unit for treatment. He is treated for opioid withdrawal with a milder opioid drug than the one he is addicted to. The substitute drug is then tapered off over the next week or two. After a wash-out period of another seven days, the patient is put on an opioid antagonist drug. The currently used antagonistic drug is Naltrexone which the patient is required to take for an extended period of time after going home. After this, even if the person happens to take heroin, Naltrexone—being the antagonist that it is—prevents the feeling of 'high' because it has blocked the opioid receptors in the brain. Since he does not feel high, there is no incentive for taking the drug. A snort or an injection now just leaves the person feeling flat because of the blockade of receptors by the antagonistic drug.

However, Naltrexone does not decrease the craving for heroin totally. Some craving persists but the person knows at an intellectual level that even if he takes it, he will not feel any pleasure. However, because craving can be compelling, chances of a patient discontinuing Naltrexone and going back to heroin are still substantial.

We often forget that what determines relapse in addictions

is not any residual withdrawal symptoms or physical discomfort as a result of not taking the drug but craving for the drug. One of the most difficult addictions to treat is nicotine addiction although nicotine has negligible withdrawal. However, the craving on giving up nicotine is strong. That is why smoking or chewing tobacco are particularly difficult habits to quit. Incidentally, Naltrexone is more effective in reducing an alcoholic's craving for alcohol than an opiate addict's craving for opioids. So, it is also used to treat alcoholism—and according to some evidence, more effectively.

B. *Harm Reduction*. The philosophy behind this treatment approach is less moralistic and more scientific and pragmatic. This approach is exactly the opposite of the abstinence-oriented treatment approach. There is no insistence upon abstinence from opioids here. In fact, very mild opioids which have very low or nil addiction potential of their own are substituted for heroin or any other opioid that the person is addicted to. This substitution takes care of craving to a great extent, and this is the reason relapse rates in addiction are lower when patients are treated with the harm reduction method rather than the abstinence method.

The following scientific rationale forms the basis of the harm reduction approach to treatment:

1. Medically pure opioid drugs, even injectable heroin, although highly habit forming, hardly ever lead to death unless an overdose is taken.

2. Addiction (as mentioned earlier), much like hypertension and arthritis, is a chronic illness. It waxes and wanes, remits and relapses. Therefore, in a large number of cases, the prognosis is guarded. Even after the patient has been off his drug of addiction, relapses do occur. It is a disease, but a chronic disease like hypertension or diabetes and not a disease like an infection,

which can be treated with a course of antibiotics and done away with.

3. Many chronic illnesses like diabetes and hypertension are genetically transmitted diseases but even then, their course can be improved by lifestyle changes and by managing environmental stress. Similarly, the course of addiction can be improved by lifestyle changes, a fulfilling job, socialization and emotionally rewarding relationships even though genetic factors are important in causation.

4. Persons who inject heroin (or other drugs) sometimes share syringes. This is because they often take drugs in small groups or in pairs. That is necessitated because heroin being illegal is difficult to obtain and pooling of resources—both logistical and financial—are required. They also need to frequently change the location where they use drugs since the fear of being caught is a constant given. If they are in a group, access to more places is possible, often a shop belonging to one of them, an isolated room on the top floor of a house which belongs to one of them or a thatch in the farm belonging to the family of a member of the group.

The availability of the drug is often unpredictable and craving strong. This results in injecting heroin as soon it is available even if only one syringe is on hand for a group. The problem is compounded by the fact that these groups are quite fluid and a young man who is injecting with a bunch of friends today could have been in another group a month back and may be injecting in a different group a month hence. He might have contacted an infection from an earlier group that he was a member of and it can be passed on to members of his current group. This is how Hepatitis-C and HIV spreads among drug addicts who then pass them on to their spouses and other sexual partners.

The harm reduction approach is an exercise in scientific humility. It acknowledges that addictions cannot be abolished from the roots because the roots lie in the human brain. The aim then is more pragmatic: to reduce as far as possible, the harms of addiction to the individual, the family and society. If a much less harmful, legally available drug can substitute a several times more harmful drug of addiction, which besides being illegal is destructive to the patient and his family, it makes sense to use it. In fact, there is nothing very novel or radical about the approach. Doctors in their routine work practice harm reduction every day. They prescribe medications to every patient, all of which could have side-effects and are harmful (to a greater or lesser extent) but are much less harmful as compared to the harms and risks associated with the disease if it is left untreated.

The specific harms caused by addiction which need to be reduced in the harm reduction approach can be listed as follows:

A lot of time and money is spent in procuring the drug. This would obviously come from the quantum of time and money which rightfully belongs to the person's family. The time spent in procuring the drug and the cycles of anticipation, intoxication and withdrawal make it difficult for the person to hold on to consistent employment.

These two factors make addiction a full-time job with no time, energy or mind space left for anything else in the person's life.

Since all these drugs are illegal, brushes with the law and actual incarceration disrupt the course of life, in addition to an ever-present apprehension of being arrested haunting him and his family members. To procure money for drugs, petty crimes born out of desperation are often resorted to and further increase the person's exposure to the criminal justice system.

In the case of addicts who inject drugs, chances of life-threatening infections like HIV and Hepatitis-C are high because of sharing of needles and syringes. In India, the number of persons affected by Hepatitis-C is eight million according to conservative estimates. Another two million have HIV infection. Injections with shared syringes, blood transfusions from suspect blood banks and unsafe sex are the three main causes of spread of both. These are fatal unless treated and together constitute a dire public health crisis, which costs the state exchequer billions of rupees.

Suppose medications were available which the patient suffering from addiction could take to treat the symptoms of withdrawal in the short term and craving in the long term. These medications would have to be cheap, at least several times cheaper than addictive drugs, easily available on prescription, which the patient could take safely without any side effects for a year or two or even longer just like the ones prescribed in treating hypertension, diabetes, psoriasis or rheumatoid arthritis.

If this was the case, the addicted person would be able to spend all the time, money and mind space now available to him with his family, which would help to mend the ruptures in family bonds caused by years of addiction and addiction behaviour. He could also hold on to a regular job without having to perpetually look over his shoulder to see if he was being followed by a policeman.

He could socialise with colleagues, relatives and friends. He would be able to go on a date or take his wife and children out. This reconnection and reintegration into society is not merely a happy outcome of the treatment of addiction, it is also the strongest protection against relapsing back into addiction. Remember the Rat Park study in which rats when offered an interesting social environment and morphine fluid chose the former? This proved that the opposite of addiction is not just abstinence from drugs but a reconnection with people.

The fact is that such treatments are available and have been available for 30-40 years, are approved by the WHO for treatment of opioid addiction and are widely used all over the world as 'opioid agonist maintenance treatment'. The medication in combination with counselling, behavioural monitoring, and provision of psychiatric, medical, or vocational services constitutes the modern treatment of addictions. Two such commonly used drugs in opioid addiction at present are Buprenorphine and Methadone. Both are weak opioid agonists, which means the two act on the same receptors in the brain as heroin or morphine. They resemble opioid drugs chemically and are their weak substitutes hence making them ideal in preventing relapses in opioid addiction. Buprenorphine is a partial agonist. While it prevents withdrawal and craving it does not give a high when taken as a tablet. Buprenorphine as a sublingual tablet is currently the most commonly used drug for maintenance treatment of opioid treatment all over the world. Buprenorphine's opioid effects increase with doses till they level off at moderate doses and after this, even with further dose increase, there is no additional effect. This 'ceiling effect' further lowers the risk of misuse, habit formation and side effects. Also, Buprenorphine being a long-acting medication, patients may not even have to take it every day. As a general rule all long-acting drugs are less habit forming.

However, in injectable form, Buprenorphine does give a high and can be addicting itself. When the drug came into use initially, there were attempts by peddlers to misuse the tablets by crushing these, mixing them with distilled water to make injections out of them. To prevent this, tablets of Buprenorphine now come as a combination of Buprenorphine and the opioid antagonist Naloxone, which is also used as an antidote for opiate overdosage. This neutralises the effect of Buprenorphine when injected thus creating no effect at all. In its tablet form containing the Buprenorphine-Naloxone combination, the Naloxone component has very poor absorption from the oral or sub-lingual route while Buprenorphine is well absorbed. As a result, instances of misuse of the combination are exceedingly low with hardly any cases of de-novo addiction.

When given to a patient of heroin addiction as a maintenance treatment, it reduces craving to a large extent. It can be said to be the drug of choice of opioid addiction at the moment. The other commonly used medication Methadone has been around since World War II. Unlike Buprenorphine, it is a complete opioid agonist and gives some feeling of a high and has some addiction potential. For this reason, unlike Buprenorphine which has now been approved as a take-home medication, Methadone is administered to the patient every day in the outpatient's clinic under direct observation.

The medication Buprenorphine (or Methadone) is used for treating withdrawal in the first phase of treatment. For this, admission to a hospital is required in about one-third of cases if the intake has been high but the majority of persons do not need admission. This part of treatment is called detoxification. This is followed by the maintenance phase at home with lower dosage of the same drug to prevent craving. This can last for a year or two or even longer but during this phase the person is able to lead a normal life, including going to work. The treatment is also called oral substitution treatment (OST), since a stronger opioid is being substituted with a very mild opioid in tablet form.

As important as the exact treatment is the way in which it is given.

A UNODC world drug report lays down the principles of treatment of addictions as follows:

a) The treatment must not just be effective, it should be easily available, accessible, attractive and appropriate.

b) It must be ethical and must not come at the cost of human rights and dignity of patients.

c) Personal data must remain confidential.

d) There must be co-ordination between the criminal justice and healthcare systems.

CHAPTER 12

On the Ground: Managing Addictions Through a Moral Lens

'Imagine if the government chased sick people with diabetes, put a tax on insulin and drove it into the black market, told doctors they couldn't treat them, then sent them to jail. If we did that, everyone would know we were crazy. Yet we do practically the same thing every day in the week to sick people hooked on drugs.'

—Billie Holiday (1915-59), US Jazz singer
who suffered from opioid addiction

Modern evidence-based treatment of addiction is available in India. Punjab alone has about 300 (about 200 in the private sector and 100 in the public sector) psychiatrists to deliver this treatment. Interestingly, many of the psychiatrists practising in Punjab are from other Indian states, some from as distant ones as Maharashtra, Karnataka and Tamil Nadu. They have relocated to Punjab over the last decade as a large number of de-addiction centres sprung up there when heroin addiction peaked in the state.

The psychiatrist to population ratio in Punjab is almost twice as compared to the national average. The state also has a very good road network which is an essential requirement for ready access to any treatment—both for first contact and follow-ups. The state government takes the issue of drug addiction seriously and is willing to allot required funding on a priority basis. This is the good news. The bad news is that society in general, the majority of the state's policy makers, politicians, bureaucrats and even some healthcare professionals still cling to their personal prejudices and moral blind spots, which stops them from viewing addictions as illnesses.

They continue to consider addictions as moral failures on the part of patients who could easily snap out of them if they really wanted to. And since patients continue to use drugs or stop using for a short while and then relapse all too frequently, this only reaffirms their belief that addicts are weak in spirit. And as their addictions make other people suffer too, addicts are labelled both weak and of bad character. Since they are 'bad' and are repeat offenders, some punishment is in order.

With the best of intentions, the Punjab Police sent out this tweet from its official handle on October 28, 2022: '#DrugAddiction reduces a man to a mindless and ridiculous thing, and creates social parasites and criminals. #SayNotoDrugs.'

This moral and stigmatising approach of society towards persons suffering from addiction makes a person and his family think hard before deciding to access treatment even when it is available. It is no surprise that only 0.5% of such persons who need treatment actually get treatment (*The Hindu*, September 26, 2019).

~

People who are prejudiced against persons suffering from addictions have several shades of opinion:

There are those who are very clear that persons with

addictions cause suffering to others including their own family members for the sake of their own pleasure, and hence are selfish people. Therefore, the only treatment they need is punishment.

For a section of the biased, persons with addiction do not deserve any treatment even for severe pains and withdrawal, which sets in when they cannot get their hands on the drug. This section of the biased argue that if you treat withdrawal every time it sets in, 'you are making things easy for addicts who might think they can indulge themselves again.' And they believe that rigours of untreated withdrawal would act as a deterrent when addicts think of taking to drugs again. Here, the understanding that addiction is an illness which remits and relapses and that uncontrollable, overpowering craving and compulsion are essential components of this illness is totally absent.

Then there is the section of the populace which accepts that some sort of treatment is required not so much for the sake of the individual but for those around him. This section conceives the patient himself as a passive recipient of treatment and not even a stakeholder in the process Also, according to them, there has to be a strong element of discipline and paternalism incorporated in the treatment (even if the patient has consented to being treated) since persons with addictions are considered 'weak', which is why they are in the situation they are in. The proponents of this approach sometimes call it tough love—a cold, authoritative approach ostensibly designed to set boundaries.

In November 2011, I had the opportunity to be part of a three-member fact-finding governmental group visiting drug rehab centres in some districts of Punjab. In just one year, sixty such centres had come up in Punjab—mainly in rural areas, to cater to the rising demand of desperate parents in the wake of the fast-spreading opioid addiction in young men. The parents were clueless about where to turn to because the young men would refuse to accompany their families to the nearest city to be treated, a process which at that time required admission to treatment centres.

Enter the newly established 'rehab centres' to solve the specific problem of pesky young men neither stopping their drug use nor willing to accept treatment. Most of these centres were run by former patients of drug addiction who claimed to understand the problem since they had themselves been there and back. Except they had not been. The claim by the owners-cum-managers of these centres having been former drug addicts turned out to be a marketing gimmick which lured the desperate parents to them. Who else, the hapless parents thought, would understand better the complexities of their son's addiction than a recovered addict? Hoping for the best, they were happy to go ahead and pay the advance, sign the affidavits and collaborate with those who ran these centres in bundling their sons in the dead of the night into a jeep belonging to the centre and carting them off. The affidavit signed by the parents was just a fig leaf for these centres.

In reality, most of the young men were eighteen and above and hence the affidavits signed by parents empowering the rehab centres to take away their sons and treat them against their wishes were worthless. But nobody ever sued, certainly not the aggrieved young men because that would have involved complaining against their parents too, which would have compounded their guilt.

But resourceful as young men are, they frequently tried to run away from the rehab centres, although only a small number succeeded. The rest were treated with 'tough love' there, which included sweeping the floor, washing clothes, helping with the cooking, washing utensils and attending yoga classes. They also had to attend lectures on the ill effects of drugs of addiction by their minders at the centres who claimed to be 'former addicts' with first-hand knowledge of addictions.

When we (the members of the fact-finding group) were escorted towards a hall beyond the reception area of a government-approved rehab centre in district Mohali, Punjab, we saw a prominent notice in Hindi at the entrance. It said, '*Apna sayana dimaag jooton ke* rack *me rakh kar aao*' (Leave your wise brain on the shoe rack at the entrance).

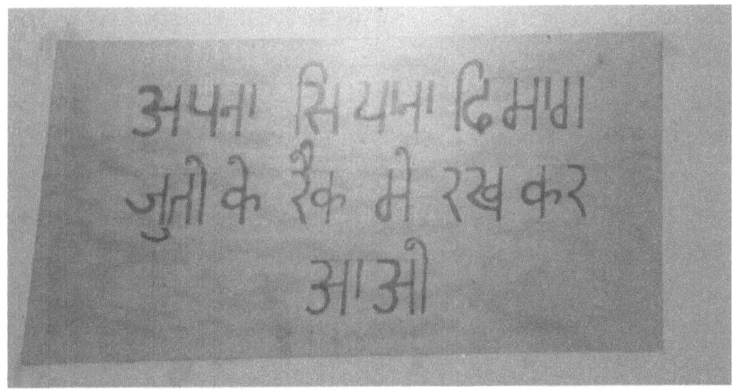

Notice pasted at the entrance of the ward of a government approved rehab centre in district Mohali, Punjab. November 2011. (Photo: Anirudh Kala)

That reminded one of us of Dante's *Inferno* and the phrase at the gates of hell, 'Abandon all hope, ye who enter here' and reiterated the absolute nature of the paternalistic approach that not just society at large but also some of the leaders, planners and officials in charge have towards persons with addiction.

The so-called 'tough love' approach has historically jostled for a place as a legitimate approach to treating persons with drug addiction. But essentially, if society does not treat diabetics with the tough love approach by locking them up and controlling what they eat, take them forcibly every morning for walks because 'it is good for them', why should this be done to persons with drug addiction? However, the fact remains that this paternalistic approach found a fertile ground in the highly patriarchal society of Punjab and the rest of India. Things are getting better but at a slow pace. India still has a long way to go when it comes to the attitude towards addictions and their treatment.

When policy makers who in the Indian setting are primarily politicians and bureaucrats, not experts, make decisions, they do so out of political compulsions. Their approach is rigidly paternalistic. Even when building treatment facilities, the single-most important element lacking is empathy. It is the system which decides the treatment, how much and for how long. The system does not provide any channel to experts or the users of the system and their families to give feedback. These primary stakeholders who are being ignored have valuable ideas which can radically improve the quality of care.

The prejudice is pervasive across all sections of society and is shared by the judiciary and the police.

The phenomenon of addiction being viewed through a moralistic prism by the Indian establishment, both at the centre and the state level, is the single largest hindrance to the benefits of scientific advances effectively reaching patients and their families. Thus, the treatment of drug addiction written about in medical and psychiatric books and scientific journals is one thing. What patients suffering from addiction get in reality after society, policy makers and the judicial system, which view things through their multiple lenses of prejudices, is something entirely different. And sometimes, even the exact opposite of what is required scientifically.

A couple of examples will suffice to point out the difference between theory and practice of treatment. They revolve around the issue of who gets treatment and who does not.

Drug addiction can be treated in Punjab only in de-addiction centres licensed by the state government under the stringent NDPS Act. Thus, the law that is applicable to smugglers also controls treatment. It is a crime under the NDPS Act even for a qualified psychiatrist to treat a patient of drug addiction outside such centres. The psychiatrist is the same, the patient is the same, the treatment is the same but it cannot be given because the surroundings are not licensed. It takes months, sometimes years, to get such a license or even to renew an already existing license. This is in spite of the fact that the Mental Health Care Act-2017 has categorically defined drug addiction as a mental illness and requires state governments to regulate treatment of addiction under the Mental Health Care Act and not under the NDPS Act, which is primarily meant to incarcerate peddlers and smugglers.

At present, no hospital other than a licensed drug de-addiction centre can treat a person with addiction, either as an outpatient or an inpatient. If a patient in need of immediate treatment is brought by the family in severe drug withdrawal to any hospital in Punjab, he cannot be treated there. The medicines for treatment are allowed to be stocked only in the licensed de-addiction centres, not in other clinics or hospitals across the state. There is no exception even for emergency overnight treatment.

As I mentioned in the previous chapter, modern treatment of opioid addiction centres around the harm reduction approach, which advocates that the treatment should concentrate on reducing harms caused by opioid addiction and not on the romantic ideal of abolishing addiction, which like hypertension or diabetes cannot be abolished. Along with counselling, it essentially involves the addicted person taking the medicine over a long period of time while being able to function as a normal member of his family and society. Society benefits because the number of people injecting drugs goes down and to that extent, the number of persons with Hepatitis-C and HIV goes down as well, leading to a saving of hundreds of millions of rupees for the public health system. On the face of it, this seems simple, straightforward and a win-win for everybody. Except, it is not, in the real world.

In Punjab, Buprenorphine has been used for about a decade-and-a-half in both government and private hospitals and has been found to be a safe and effective medicine. It is included in the WHO list of essential medicines. In September 2022, it was included in the National List of Essential Medicines and its price reduced to make it easily affordable. In spite of this, it continues to be a highly restricted drug. Buprenorphine is one of the medicines listed under the NDPS Act, which if found on a person without a prescription or other authorization, results in the person's arrest and prosecution. The person can be sentenced under the NDPS for a duration of time, which is proportionate to the number of tablets he is carrying.

Thus, while the medications for treatment are available as are psychiatrists qualified to treat addiction, patients' access to treatment has been patchy over the years because of two administrative hindrances:

i) Treatment for addiction can be done only in specific standalone licensed de-addiction centres. The process of licensing takes a long time and it is opaque.

Even a qualified psychiatrist cannot treat a patient of addiction as part of his psychiatric practice outside such a centre, it being a criminal offence. The standalone nature of the treatment facility adds to the stigma of drug addiction. This then acts as a barrier to free access to treatment because patients and their families are wary of being seen by others at a de-addiction centre.

ii) The specific medications used for treatment of addiction like Buprenorphine are supplied only to licensed de-addiction centres. If a psychiatrist who runs a licensed de-addiction centre is carrying Buprenorphine in his car to his own satellite clinic for use by bonafide patients suffering from addiction and is intercepted on the way, he is arrested and proceeded against under the NDPS Act. Four psychiatrists under such circumstances have been arrested in Punjab and incarcerated for several months. All of them are currently on bail and fighting their legal battles.

Eleanora Fagan, better known as Billie Holiday (1915-59), was a popular American jazz singer who won four Grammy awards, all posthumously, and has been hailed as 'perhaps the greatest female jazz vocalist there ever was.' During her lifetime, she was hounded by the police for her opioid addiction. Her apartment was raided many times and she was jailed twice for possessing narcotics for personal use. Doctors who tried to treat her were threatened and she was denied treatment. Holiday wrote in her memoir shortly before her death, 'Imagine if the government chased sick people with diabetes, put a tax on insulin and drove it into the black market, told doctors they couldn't treat them, then sent them to jail.'

She added, 'If we did that, everyone would know we were crazy. Yet, we do practically the same thing every day of the week to sick people hooked on drugs.' What Holiday wrote about treatment and policy-making in America six decades back continues to hold true in present-day India, particularly so in Punjab.

The process of treating patients within the four walls of licensed de-addiction centres is governed less by evidence-based medicine and more by arbitrary rules framed under the NDPS Act. At the heart of the matter is the discomfort of those in charge about the principle of a harm reduction strategy like Buprenorphine. Their discomfort stems from the fact that Buprenorphine is itself an opioid. It is a much weaker one compared to opium or heroin which it replaces with negligible addictiveness, but it still is a distant chemical cousin of heroin or opium. And society too finds this difficult to absorb notwithstanding the fact that the treatment is backed by years of research, approved by the WHO as the standard treatment of opioid addiction and is used as a safe and effective outpatient-based treatment all over the world.

But politicians, bureaucrats and the media are doubtful. They view it as a treatment which substitutes one addiction with another. 'A person was addicted to an opioid drug before, and he is addicted to an opioid drug now. What has changed?' they ask. They accuse doctors of profiting off of it, thus vilifying the treatment process in an indignant moral sweep. The prejudice, bias and exclusion with which society treats mental illness in general is on display with even more intensity when dealing with the treatment of addiction. Unfortunately, psychiatrists who treat addiction are not just stigmatized but are also accused of peddling drugs to addicts in the garb of treatment because the argument is that addicts need discipline, and not treatment with medicines, which are of a similar nature as that of the drugs which the patient was addicted to, to start with.

Headlines demonising the treatment of addiction and castigating psychiatrists for using OST have appeared regularly over the last decade in newspapers in Punjab. Even reputed and otherwise balanced publications have been vilifying doctors for using a treatment which is an evidence-based one used worldwide. An aging chief minister of Punjab once admonished a delegation of psychiatrists who had gone to meet him to request liberalized rules for the treatment of addiction. He compared their request to allowing opium vends to be set up at every street corner much like liquor vends. The state health minister in an interview to a newspaper took it upon himself to declare that patients of opioid addiction should be given their medication only while they are admitted in wards and not as outpatients, since it was a 'strong medicine' and may be misused by their friends and relatives who may then get addicted to it and create fresh problems for the government by adding to the existing number of addicts.

Both these statements were made off the cuff in the absence of any evidence. But the police took a cue from the health minister's widely reported statement. In the following week, two psychiatrists treating addiction were arrested for the 'offence' of possession of tablets of de-addiction medicine. The next day's headlines said, 'Psychiatrists protest arrest of two colleagues, stop prescribing drugs to addicts' and 'Psychiatrists acting as drug peddlers.'

This sent a chilling message to the mental health professionals of the state who stopped prescribing Buprenorphine out of fear. So, during the exceptionally grey and foggy winter of 2014, patients of heroin addiction in Punjab had no recourse to medication. Satyen Sharma, a psychiatrist from Punjab, presented an account of that period at a conference in a paper titled, 'The Cold Turkey State.' Many patients who reported for treatment in the subsequent months reported having had gone back to heroin in that winter of 2014, because heroin 'was more easily available than the treatment'.

Steps like these destroy the credibility of the process of

treatment by demonising it. The families who are already unsure about whether to go for treatment back away. The doctors who treat addiction in Punjab are not allowed to treat it as they would treat other illnesses, drawing from their training, experience, latest research published in medical journals or treatment guidelines framed by their professional organizations. They have to treat addiction according to a Standard Operating Procedures (SOP) issued by the state government the essence of which is 'prescribe as little as possible', whatever the science.

The SOP is a managerial rather than a medical concept. The current SOP is not based on any scientific evidence and has not been published in any peer-reviewed medical journal. It states among other things that opioid maintenance treatment should not be used for addiction to opium husk or 'low-quality' opium and should be used for only heroin or high-quality opium. This recommendation flies in the face of logic and is not mentioned in any medical textbook or research paper on opioid addiction. It is as unreasonable as laying down a rule that alcoholism caused by drinking beer should be treated with a milder and lesser dose of medication than alcoholism caused by whiskey.

In 2017, the WHO issued recommendations that *policy makers must not place restrictions on dose levels and duration of treatment*. However, doctors treating addictions in Punjab keep receiving letters from the government demanding to know the dosage and duration of treatment of patients.

The government also asks how many patients have been weaned off the medication, indicating that stopping treatment early is better. This unseemly hurry driven purely by morality is the reason of many relapses and would increase, not decrease, overdosage deaths. It would also increase the morbidity and mortality associated with HIV and Hepatitis-C infections along with the associated increase in public health expenditure.

It is bizarre that while the government does not pursue endocrinologists to give less insulin to patients of diabetes and to stop treatment early, it hounds psychiatrists to do so when it comes to treating addiction.

The common thread in all the rules and circulars is the same: be as tight-fisted with medication in treating addictions as possible. The premise has no scientific basis. It is based solely on the prejudice against all addictions and people suffering from them. While the WHO insists that there should be minimal interference by administrators in the protocols of addiction treatment, in Punjab, all the district de-addiction committees are headed not by doctors but by deputy commissioners. And since the treatment of addiction seems to be 'common sense' to an outsider, common sense, not science, dominates the discourse.

Thus, on June 10, 2022, the deputy commissioner of Muktsar in Punjab called a meeting of the district de-addiction committee in the wake of six overdosage deaths in the previous month, which was featured prominently in newspapers.

Some of the decisions taken at the meeting were:

1. The de-addiction centres should publicise widely that treatment is available at specific places in the district.

2. The doctors should reduce the dose of Buprenorphine as far as possible.

3. A weekly report of results of such efforts by doctors should be sent to the district civil surgeon's office.

4. A detailed list of all the patients who come in for treatment for opioid addiction, including their names, address and phone numbers in Excel format be sent to the district headquarters. And biometric identification of patients had to be done before giving them the medicine.

Nobody explained the logic behind publicising the

availability of de-addiction medicines on the one hand while advocating that patients should be given as little of the medicine as possible on the other. And nobody asked the question that if addiction is indeed a disease like diabetes, would the deputy commissioner of a district press upon doctors to decrease the dose of anti-diabetic drugs, have diabetic patients biometrically identified before giving them medicines and circulate lists of their personal details. The problem is that neither society nor politicians and administrators actually think addiction is a real disease. Hence the 'common sense, disciplinarian' approach.

In a remarkably similar counter-intuitive measure, the deputy commissioner of Gurdaspur issued an order to ASHA health workers to conduct a survey of persons with drug addiction in their locations and send the lists of all such persons to the government including each person's name, phone number and address. Addiction is a disease and the preparation and circulation of such lists is deeply stigmatizing. It leads to societal exclusion which worsens the addiction besides being a violation of the person's right to privacy.

If the intention is to treat them, let everybody know of the facilities being provided by the state and allow the persons with addiction to approach these facilities voluntarily. It is understandable that deputy commissioners in charge of all the departments in a district would not know the intricacies of each department, particularly when it comes to medical science. For that reason alone, medical treatment should not be micro-managed by administrators and politicians.

~

The press has done more than its fair share in vilifying the treatment of addiction. In a recent editorial titled, 'Hooked on De-addiction Pill,' by the otherwise reputed *Tribune*, the paper went on to lament, 'Many patients, during their journey of ridding themselves of habit-forming substances, often find themselves sinking deeper into the morass as they become addicted to the very medicine that was meant to cure them.' This is very much like saying that patients of type 1 diabetes are addicted to insulin, 'the very medicine that is meant to cure them.' Or pointing fingers at the treatment of hypertension, which stipulates that patients have to take tablets for years. This lazy and sensationalist approach simply fails to recognise the fatal and debilitating effects of not taking insulin or blood pressure medicines or Buprenorphine.

There is a deliberate reluctance to face the fact that all treatments have side effects, but we still take them because the harmful effects of not taking them far outweigh the risks of taking them.

Addiction implies an out-of-control use that leads to alcohol or a drug determining the priorities of the individual. Do addicted persons and families on treatment sometimes feel they are stuck on Buprenorphine for months or sometimes, years? Yes. But the fact is that these persons are unlikely to die from an overdose, end up in jail, develop HIV or Hepatitis-C, have marital problems or lose their jobs, which would have likely happened had they not been receiving the treatment.

~

Like a moral hawk, the Punjab state health department's office controls and monitors in real time every prescription given to all patients of addiction through a high-tech online software system. The system records every patient's name, father's name, address, photo and Aadhaar card. Every time a doctor in a de-addiction centre in the state sees a new or a follow up patient he must log into this system and enter the number of tablets of medication prescribed. If the treatment is dispensed for more than seven days, justification must be provided. Medicines cannot be prescribed for more than fourteen days in any case. The system does not allow medicines to be prescribed for more than two weeks even if the patient is planning to travel abroad or is recovering from a surgery. The fear of the medicine being misused drives this decision, ignoring the fact that the medicine, in contrast to the heroin that the patient was taking, is far safer and has negligible addictive potential.

The only instances of 'misuse' that have been proven are cases where a person who is unable to go to a centre on a particular day to fetch his medicine because of either work or family commitments borrowing tablets from a friend who is also being treated for his own addiction. When the person is able to go and get his own medication, he returns that many tablets to his friend.

Another hurdle psychiatrists in Punjab face is that prescribing offline is punishable with cancellation of license and prosecution under the NDPS Act. So, whenever the central registry website faces a technical glitch and stops working, psychiatrists across the state (in the government as well as private de-addiction centres) stop working and patients are asked to wait. Although there are some provisions to prescribe offline for the limited time when the online system is not working, such is the fear that it is considered safer to wait.

The history of treatment of addiction in Punjab is replete with episodes of one step forward, two backward every few months. This damages whatever progress has been made by the government itself.

Confidentiality is an integral part of the treatment process whatever the illness and nature of treatment. This becomes crucial when the nature of an illness is already stigmatising—

and society has deep prejudices against mental illnesses and drug addictions. Individual doctors are sworn to keep identifying details of patients confidential as part of an ethical code which is enforced by the Medical Council of India and patients trust the doctors about maintaining confidentiality. However, the government office staff have no such ethical responsibility. When a patient with addiction comes to know that every time he enters a treatment facility, all his identifying data is recorded on a system by the health department, there is a deep sense of betrayal.

The father of a young man put it like this, 'If I had a daughter of marriageable age, I know what I would have done while selecting a match for her. I would have tried to find out from Chandigarh if the boy had ever taken treatment for heroin addiction since it is so common. I hear it's all there on a government computer. And I am sure when I think of marrying my son off, the girls' parents would have the same worry and might want to find out these details about my son.'

Their fears are well founded because in the past, the state police had attempted to pressurise doctors to share the names and addresses of their patients being treated for addiction, saying they wanted to interrogate patients to ask about the source of their supply in order to arrest peddlers. Doctors pushed back and their associations resisted citing confidentiality. *The Indian Express* dated July 17, 2015 featured a blistering editorial titled 'Bad habit: Punjab police's attempts to extract patient records from de-addiction centres put such programmes at risk.'

The editorial said, 'In what constitutes a breathtakingly obdurate and insensitive attempt at police work, Punjab's cops have reportedly been asking the state's de-addiction centres to hand over data on patients. Apparently, the police want such centres to release details such as names, addresses and telephone numbers. Perhaps the police believe that speaking to addicts can help them trace the dealers and suppliers of the drugs, so action can be taken against them. But they must also be aware that their demands represent a substantial overreach of authority and could be actively harmful. If rehabilitation centres were to divulge this information, it would not just constitute a massive breach of privacy, it would also undermine trust in these places, thus endangering these programmes in a state that sorely needs them.'

It is not that there has been a complete absence of rational and sane phases. There certainly have been. But no policy about the treatment of opiate addiction has been institutionalized yet. Among the hundreds of thousands of documents, e-mails, memos and orders generated in the offices of the Punjab government over the last few decades about drug addiction and its treatment, all steps have been ad-hoc.

The problem with such ad-hocism is that even the progressive steps are highly subjective and individualistic in philosophy. They keep changing when a new health minister or health secretary takes charge. The new incumbents bring in their own moral baggage which in turn affects the way drug addiction is viewed—either as a medical disorder or a moral failing. The ad-hoc policy which springs from their thinking sets back progress that has been made.

The government of Punjab has no institutional memory about drug addiction in the state. It even forgets the many laudable steps it has taken over the years and that is a pity. As of now, the state government is trying to liberalise access to medication in the government sector with an emphasis on outpatient rather than inpatient treatment, but there is no guarantee that this would outlast the next round of transfers of government officials or a change in government after the next elections.

CHAPTER 13

The Liberalization Debate

Former US president Richard Nixon launched America's War on Drugs in 1971, a campaign aiming to ban all habit-forming chemicals *other than caffeine, alcohol and nicotine.* This 'war' was adopted by the rest of the world after most countries were coaxed, cajoled and arm-twisted by America using diplomatic channels and US aid as leverage to sign the relevant UN multilateral treaties. However, some countries like China which had their own opium use problem did readily co-operate with the US. The UN treaties in turn legally bound the signee governments to declare it a criminal act in their countries to produce, possess, trade and consume all drugs except for medical and scientific purposes.

The drugs prohibited under the UN Single Convention in 1961 are products of three plants—opium, cannabis and cocoa, or are synthetic analogues of these plant products. The latter category would include drugs like heroin, methamphetamine and LSD.

In addition, in 1971, at the UN Convention on Psychotropic Substances in Vienna, the manufacture, transport and sale of many pharmaceutical formulations such as amphetamine-type stimulants, barbiturates, benzodiazepines and psychedelics for uses other than medical and scientific purposes were also made a crime all over the world.

The primary purpose of these UN conventions is not altruistic concern for the health of humankind but to reduce illegal drug trade into the USA by enforcing harsh drug laws not just within the USA but all over the world. From the American point the reasoning was, 'What is the use of prohibiting drugs in the USA when these can be brought to the country from anywhere in the world?'

This international arrangement even entitles the US state apparatus to use its military to prevent these drugs from entering America. The War on Drugs in the global context thus includes a set of drug policies that are intended to criminalise certain designated drugs that the United Nations has banned at America's behest.

The term 'War on Drugs' was popularized by the media after Nixon declared illicit drugs 'public enemy number one' in a message to the US Congress in 1971. That message also included suggestions about devoting more federal resources to 'the prevention of creation of new addicts and the rehabilitation of those who are addicted', but the part pertaining to prevention and rehabilitation did not receive as much public attention as the term 'War on Drugs'.

It is important to remember that according to the UN conventions and the country-specific laws, which sprung from these global treaties, there is now no such thing as legal recreational drug use on the planet. All drug use has to be only for medical or research purposes.

We know that a vast majority of people who use drugs are not harmed by them. Only a small minority are. This has been borne out by many international studies including India's National Drug Survey, 2019. Even in the case of the highly addictive group of drugs like opioids, out of 2% of Indians who use these, 0.26% are addicted. In the case of the cannabis group of drugs like weed and ganja, the figures are 2.83% and 0.25%. The statement that a vast majority of drug users are not harmed by drugs is valid worldwide not because the drugs themselves are harmless—that they certainly are not—but because responsible drug use is the norm rather than the exception.

A 1991 US population survey suggested that about one in four people who used heroin had become dependent at some point of time before they were interviewed. The other three had not. And heroin is chemically one of the most addictive drugs known to us.

This is in no way meant to convey that since there is a 75% chance one could take heroin a few times and then leave it without getting addicted and can safely experiment with it. *Heroin addiction destroys individuals and wrecks families.* Even 25% is a very high number. I have cited this statistic only to drive home an essential point in understanding addiction. The chemical qualities of a drug, any drug, are not the only factor which leads to addiction and banning the drug is not a solution but a problem in itself. Those of us who drink do so to relax. We also use alcohol as a social facilitator. And most people who smoke weed do so because they like the alternate experience it provides for a few hours.

However, all we hear about in public discussions on drugs are casualties. This drives official policy which then governs, criminalises and penalises all of users by making mere consumption a crime too.

If enacting harsh laws and sending some people to jail could prevent the damage to individuals, families and society, most people would agree that the long-drawn War on Drugs makes sense. In that case, to expect all users (even casual ones) to totally abstain from drugs would be reasonable, and sending those who still used drugs to jail would be justified.

Afterall, when governments institute a law that declares driving under the influence (DUI) of alcohol a crime, it is nobody's logic that every person who drives after drinking causes accidents. In fact, we know that many people who drive under the effect of alcohol manage to reach their destinations safely. But since there is evidence that alcohol impairs co-ordination and slows down reflexes and having such a law does lower traffic accidents and saves lives, the law banning driving after drinking makes complete sense. Similarly, the law about using seat belts while driving or riding automobiles and wearing helmets while driving two-wheelers does not presuppose that every person who does not do so has a fatal accident. But again, there is strong evidence suggesting seat belts and helmets decrease the overall incidence of deaths and disability. This evidence makes these laws logical and in the public interest.

However, do we have such evidence regarding the War on Drugs and its enforcement through the criminal justice system? Does prohibition and banning drugs decrease the number of deaths and scale of misery caused by addiction at all? Trillions of dollars have been spent on trying to win this War, and it has resulted in the imprisonment of millions of people worldwide in the process. It is high time to ask, 'Is this working?'

In an article titled 'Global Patterns of Opioid Use and Dependence: Harms to Populations, Interventions, and Future Action', the reputed medical journal *The Lancet* reported that during 2017, 40.5 million people worldwide were addicted to opioids and 109,500 died from opioid overdose. Out of all the overdosage deaths which occurred in the world, 43% were in the USA which only has 4.27% of the world's population.

The severity of the opioid problem reduced adult life

expectancy in the USA for three consecutive years (2014-17), a first since 1964. During 2017, globally, prevalence of opioid dependence was 510 persons per 100,000 population. The country with the highest estimated prevalence in 2017 was the USA at 1,347 per 100,000.

The USA, the global leader of the War on Drugs has the largest and the most richly funded Drug Enforcement Authority (DEA) in the world. Americans constitute 4.2% of the world population but the country has 20% of the world's prison population, a large part of which is thanks to the War on Drugs. Out of every 100,000 of the population, 639 Americans are in jail—the highest rate in the world. It still has a concentration of persons addicted to drugs almost three times more than the global average and a number of overdosage deaths ten times the global average. Surely, this is enough proof for the world to pause and consider the very likely possibility that we are losing this so-called War on Drugs because maybe we got it all wrong.

We should be 'managing' drugs rather than waging a War. Wars are waged by one country against another; whoever heard of a war against inanimate objects or against one's own people!

Jeffrey Miron, an economist at Harvard University, estimated about ten years ago that ending the War on Drugs would infuse 76.8 billion dollars into the US economy in one year. The government would save $41.3 billion that is being spent on drug enforcement and keeping people in prison, and would additionally mop up $46.7 billion in taxes if drug sales were regulated like alcohol.

A total of thirty-seven million nonviolent drug offenders have been incarcerated since President Nixon declared the War on Drugs. A total of $121 billion was spent to arrest these offenders and $450 billion to keep them in jails. In the USA, the government spends one million dollars for every five people it arrests, prosecutes and convicts of mid-level drug offences. 90% of the money spent on drug policy by the US government goes to policing and punishment and only 10% to treatment and prevention.

The counter argument that some proponents of the War on Drugs put forward goes like this: the fact that America is spending so much money and effort on this war is precisely because it has such a high prevalence of drug addiction and sky-high numbers of overdosage deaths in the first place. The implication here is that but for the War, these numbers would have been even higher, and the concerted warlike effort is indeed yielding results to that extent.

There is no proof to support this counter argument. But let us focus on some 'outlier' countries which have in the last few years reversed course by liberalising their drug laws and see if their world has come crashing down as a result. All evidence so far suggests that it has not. On the contrary, the individuals, families and societies in these countries have heaved a collective sigh of relief and have no intention of restarting that War. It is important to stress that advocates of liberalising drug laws do not ask that all drugs should be freely available on street corners to be taken by whosoever wants to. This libertarian access is not what serious thinkers support.

Three terms are commonly used to clarify this:

Liberalising a drug is a broad concept which pertains to making the drug laws liberal and includes various shades of opinion.

Decriminalization means to stop treating both the consumption of a drug and possession of small quantities for personal use as criminal offences. The production and sale still remain illegal and in the hands of smugglers and gangsters. The benefit to society here is that the huge sums of money spent on arresting, prosecuting and jailing hundreds of thousands of people found in possession of small amounts of a drug can be saved. This money can be spent on treating persons with addiction and educating the general population about the ill effects of drugs.

Legalising a drug, however, implies that not only are the consumption and possession of small amounts of that particular drug no longer criminal offences, but even their production and sale are allowed under government regulations. Standardized quality of a drug is available to adults in a fixed quantity at intervals at licensed stores. Thus, production and sale are taken away from gangsters and peddlers and brought under government supervision. (Alcohol and tobacco are legalized drugs in most parts of the world including India. However, in many Islamic countries and some Indian states such as Gujarat and Bihar, alcohol is illegal).

Legalization has three distinct benefits over and above those of liberalization:

a) The tax on the now legal drug (like the one on alcohol and tobacco at present) will help the government earn a substantial amount as revenue.

b) When a drug is legalized, gangsters and smugglers vanish and their gang wars over territories stop. This leads to a huge improvement in the overall law and order situation and brings in further savings to the state, which spends enormous sums to maintain law and order.

c) Many of the harmful effects of drugs like overdosage deaths are because of adulteration. The predictable quality when a drug is legalized takes care of this problem and hands over some degree of control to the person who is using the drug. Moreover, if a user wants to taper off his intake, he can do that more easily as compared to the situation at present. Right now, the user has no clue about the quality of the drug and hence cannot correctly calibrate his dose even when he wants to stop taking it over a period of time.

The basic principle of liberalization is pragmatism. Since drugs cannot be wished away the effort should be to minimise their harm to individuals and to society as far as possible.

The benefits of decriminalization and legalization can be better understood if we look at what several countries have achieved with their pragmatic initiatives.

Portugal: Portugal is known as the *first country in the world to have decriminalized all drugs* from cannabis to cocaine to heroin. This happened in 2001. The bloodless 'Carnation Revolution' in 1974 liberated the country from decades-old authoritarian rule and after a process of stabilization, the nation started the process of writing a new constitution. The far sightedness of the new regime lay in the fact that on the drug front they decided to have a radically new policy although it took time for national consensus to build.

Portugal in the 1980s had cannabis and cocaine use which was low by international standards, but heroin use was much higher than the world average. The government was desperate and having had no past experience of dealing with this crisis, went ahead and followed what the rest of the world was doing—join the international War on Drugs and follow its norms of crack down, criminalise and incarcerate. Portugal took to it like a new convert. But to their puzzlement, heroin use rose further as did the number of people infected with AIDs as a result of intravenous heroin use. By the late 90s, it was difficult to find an unaffected family even among the well to do.

The government formed an independent panel of nine doctors and judges with an academician as its chairperson whose remit was to come up with a plan to pull the country out of the morass. They were given complete freedom to think afresh which meant they could come up with unconventional ideas no other country could.

The first thing they focused on was that the largest chunk of the population of drug users was not made up of addicts. They were the people who used drugs discriminately and could be your work friends, people with whom you commuted to town daily or your neighbours who were going about their business in a perfectly normal fashion. The committee decided that the state need not concern itself with this large population except for spreading awareness among them about safe drug use.

The second group was smaller but more crucial: people who were addicted to drugs. It was the opinion of the members that the criminalization, arrests and incarceration of addicts was the single most important hindrance in the treatment of addiction. The committee recommended, 'Instead of striving towards an unachievable perfection like zero drug use, intake of drugs should be decriminalized, and drug users should be treated as full members of society instead of being treated as pariahs and criminals. The money spent on arresting, trying and incarcerating addicts should be diverted to educating kids about drugs and treating drug addicts.'

The Portuguese parliament, to the surprise of many international observers, actually debated the committee recommendations thoroughly. Many members of the public were already convinced after observing their own family members that drug addicts were ill and needed treatment rather than punishment. The Portuguese parliament in 2001 passed a law decriminalising the use of *all* drugs without exception. And possession of a small number of drugs—up to one's ten-day usage was no longer a crime. However, selling drugs would still be a crime as in other countries.

Some may find this logically troubling in the sense that if the users are using the drugs legally, they must be buying these from somebody who is selling illegally. This also means that supply of drugs remains in the hands of gangs and cartels. However, it was wise to keep it that way because Portugal wanted to work within the boundaries of the UN conventions. Legalising and regulating sales would have meant that Portugal would have become the first ever outlier country, inviting a crackdown and a slew of international sanctions.

Does this mean that if India wants to do exactly what Portugal did twenty years back about decriminalising consumption and possession for personal use, it can go ahead without falling foul of the multilateral treaties it has signed? Yes, it absolutely can if it really wants to. The United Nations Convention Against Illicit Traffic in Narcotic Drugs and Psychotropic Substances of 1988 gives a certain leeway to countries as far as personal use is concerned. Article 3.2 of the convention stipulates:

'Subject to its constitutional principles and the basic concepts of its legal system, each country shall adopt such measures as may be necessary to establish as a criminal offence under its domestic law, when committed intentionally, the possession, purchase or cultivation of narcotic drugs or psychotropic substances for personal consumption.' Hence, as far as personal consumption itself is concerned individual countries can pass internal laws like Portugal did in 2001.

However, the extent of reforms undertaken by Portugal go far beyond decriminalising use and possession of small amounts. The reform led to the policy of leaving non-addicted users alone other than providing safety advice to them. These were the crucial first steps but these were not enough according to the expert panel. According to Johann Hari, 'Portugal took the big lumbering machinery of the drug war and turned it into an equally big, active machine to establish a drug peace.' The major impact of decriminalization was that the government was now free to formulate other policies. In the US, 90% of the money spent on drug policy is spent on policing and jails and 10% on treatment and prevention. In Portugal, after 2001, it has been almost exactly the other way around.

The police in Portugal do not come looking for drug users and do not erect road barricades to search youngsters' scooters and backpacks like the Punjab police did during the whole of 2014 (and continue to do so even today quite often).

In Portugal, unless you are seen blatantly smoking a drug in public or if you are involved in a street fight and then are searched and a drug for personal use is recovered, the police will leave you alone. In the instances of public smoking or of a small amount of drug being found on your person, you will be issued a ticket like a parking ticket, which will not appear on your criminal record. The ticketed person has to appear before a Dissuasion Commission the next day where a psychologist will talk to him for about an hour to assess if he is a casual user or addicted to drugs. Only then is it decided if you need treatment. There are many who use drugs only once a month or once a week. They do it because they like it.

In such cases, a psychologist will advise them about safe drug use, tell them to never use alone because they might suffer an adverse reaction. Students will be warned that cannabis can affect their concentration. After this, some pamphlets about the adverse effects of drugs are handed out and people are free to go. Sometimes, there is a nominal fine, particularly if the person has come in more than once, but even then, there is no criminal record. In case you are found guilty of unsafe use like by sharing needles, you will be directed to the needle sharing programmes.

As far as the rest of the 10% of drug users who are addicted goes, a sociologist refers them to the nearest treatment facility. Treatment is voluntary and free. The emphasis is on talking to patients to build trust, then formal counselling and medication. The important thing is that after the treatment phase, the handholding continues, and the person gets help all the way in starting afresh and building a new life. As connections with family and society become stronger and rewarding, the connection with drugs becomes weaker, less rewarding and over time, wither away.

The government gives a one-year tax break to anybody who employs a recovering addict. In many cases, employers retain these employees for longer because they find most of them bright, hardworking and motivated. Co-operative societies of persons recovering from drug addiction have been formed and some of these even run companies. The peer group here is honest in its expectations because everybody knows what addiction is all about. There would be some relapses under the best of circumstances and if one member of the group relapses the rest of the group sees him through the bad patch.

If there are persons who need substitution treatment, Methadone vans with social workers are sent into communities at fixed timings where people can take a dose of Methadone in plastic cups and socialise unselfconsciously in the open because persons with addiction are no longer stigmatized. The social workers in the vans also listen to persons who are still on drugs and try to convince them to shift from injecting heroin to snorting because the latter only rarely causes overdosage. The message is that of acceptance and not exclusion.

For persons with addictions who are living on the streets or in abandoned housing projects, there is a different set of dedicated teams, while earlier, the police would manhandle them and arrest them. Persons with addiction look forward to the arrival of these teams because they represent society reaching out to them rather than casting them away. The outcome measures of all these radical drug reforms have been studied objectively by impartial international bodies.

Whenever drug laws are liberalized, a slight increase in overall use, mostly casual use, is expected and that did happen in Portugal. The overall drug use rose from 3.4 to 3.7% of the population. But Portugal ten years after decriminalization was still the ninth lowest among all European countries in cannabis use and the fifth lowest in amphetamine and Ecstasy use.

Moreover, the hardcore indices of addiction improved significantly. *The crimes related to drug addiction no longer happen because a large number of users are on Methadone or other treatments.* Before the liberalization of the drug policy critics in Portugal as well as in America and in some European countries predicted a doomsday scenario. The critics in the conservative and largely Catholic society of Portugal said it would open the doors wide to 'drug tourists' and exacerbate Portugal's already serious drug problem. The country had the highest level of hard-drug use in Europe at that time.

Whenever decriminalization is proposed for consumption and possession for personal use, the major fear bandied about is that teenage use will increase exponentially and spiral out of control. Since a teenager's brain is still developing, the fear does have a legitimate basis. However, in Portugal no such increase was seen. On the contrary, heroin use by teenagers went down from 2.5 to 1.8%. The credit for this largely goes to school awareness workshops conducted by students themselves under the supervision of teachers.

The number of problematic drug users has halved as has injecting drug use. Overdosage death figures are down significantly and the proportion of addiction-caused AIDS among all patients of AIDS has decreased from 52 to 32%. 'Judging by every metric, decriminalization in Portugal has been a resounding success,' wrote Glenn Greenwald, attorney and author of the Cato Institute report (2009). 'It has enabled the Portuguese government to manage and control the drug problem far better than virtually every other western country.'

Portugal's neighbours, Spain and Italy, are still waging the War on Drugs. Portugal is the only country out of the three where there has been a decline in problematic drug use. The people of Portugal are now completely invested in the drug policy having seen the dividends society reaped.

The Cato report states that between 2001 and 2006 in Portugal the rates of lifetime use of any illegal drug among seventh through ninth graders fell from 14.1% to 10.6%. Drug use in older teens also declined. Lifetime heroin use among 16 to 18-year-olds fell from 2.5% to 1.8% (although there was a slight increase in marijuana use in that age group). New HIV infections in drug users fell by 17% between 1999 and 2003, and deaths related to heroin and similar drugs were cut by more than half. In addition, the number of people on Methadone and Buprenorphine treatment for drug addiction rose to 14,877 from 6,040 after decriminalization, and the money saved on enforcement allowed for increased funding of drug-free treatment.

The Cato report has its critics led (predictably) by the White House in the USA. In 2010, the White House published a fact sheet titled 'Drug Decriminalization in Portugal: Challenges and Limitations'. This is critical of the report on statistical grounds. It says that the Cato report does not discuss the statistical significance of the data shifts it highlights. Further, White House fact sheet notes, 'the report attributes favourable trends as a direct result of decriminalization without acknowledging, for example, the decline in drug-related deaths that began prior to decriminalization. It refers to the statistics compiled by the European Monitoring Centre for Drugs and Drug Addiction (EMCDDA) which indicate that between 2001 and 2007, lifetime prevalence rates for use of cannabis, cocaine, amphetamines, ecstasy and LSD have risen for the Portuguese general population (ages 15-64) and for the 15-34 age group.' However, even the fact sheet does not contradict the finding that heroin use has come down after decriminalization. In fact, it confirms that people now prefer less harmful drugs.

The fact sheet concludes that even if there were benefits of Portugal's new and liberal drug policy these may not happen in other countries. The reason: gains could have happened because the situation in Portugal was so bad before liberalization that things could only get better! However, if the US policy makers were so convinced about decriminalization of a drug leading to bad outcomes, it is pertinent to ask why the US has followed suit at least about cannabis and not just decriminalized the drug but legalised it for recreational use in twenty-one states (where it is available in stores), which is a step far more radical than the one Portugal took.

According to an end-of-the-year CBS News Poll, support for legal pot hit a new high in 2019 in the US, with 65% of adults saying marijuana should be legal. And, for the first time, a majority of Republicans (56%) favoured legalising marijuana.

Meanwhile experts and the people of Portugal continue to be satisfied with the results of their new drug policy. Since decriminalization, Portugal has had two governments of—one left, two right—and nobody has even talked of going back to the War on Drugs.

Switzerland: In the 1980s, injectable heroin use in Switzerland had assumed the proportion of a full-blown public health crisis.

This was associated with approximately 500 HIV cases per million people, the highest rate then in western Europe. Half of all new cases of HIV transmission were linked to heroin injection by persons addicted to heroin and at that time, no specific treatment of HIV infection was available and hence, mortality rates were very high. Both at the individual and the societal level there was growing panic about contact with drug users who ended up being shunned socially. A 1975 law had enforced prohibition of drugs with vigour.

This law favoured total abstinence from all drugs and led to a large number of arrests and mandatory registration of all drug users resulting in even more stigmatization and isolation of persons with addiction. Harm reduction measures like needles and syringes programmes were rejected and licenses for Methadone substitution clinics were made very hard to get. The state response failed, with heroin injections and HIV figures rising sharply. Zurich was particularly affected, with the number of people who injected drugs in the city growing exponentially from 4,000 at the time of the 1975 law, to 10,000 in 1985, 20,000 in 1988 and 30,000 in 1992.

The Zurich city authorities in a bold move dedicated a separate area where persons with addiction were allowed to use drugs without it being illegal. The space became known as 'Needle Park'. Health services and the needle programme could be now targeted at a specific location. Between 1988 and 1992, the project responded to 6,700 overdosage episodes, vaccinated thousands for Hepatitis-B, and distributed ten million sterile syringes. Needle Park was closed down abruptly after four years owing to complaints from the people living around the area and the HIV crisis worsened once again.

Switzerland rolled out the Swiss Heroin Assisted Treatment (HAT) programme in 1994, for persons with addiction to heroin injections for whom nothing else had worked. This was a resounding success.

The three requirements before one could be enrolled in a HAT clinic were:

1. You must be above 18.

2. You must have undergone at least two other treatment programmes earlier without any success.

3. You must surrender your driving license.

Patients were required to attend a clinic once or twice a day, were seen by a specialist and prescribed heroin. They could use their prescriptions only on site and injections were given under medical supervision. The basic premise here was that pure heroin, given with clean syringes under medical supervision is relatively harmless, and when given to heroin addicts *in whom all other treatments have failed* is beneficial to persons with addiction as well as to society. The idea was to combine the advantages of:

a) Prescribed dose of heroin of known strength and purity, free from contaminants and adulterants, and used with clean injecting equipment thus preventing HIV and hepatitis infections.

b) Regular access to services and supervised use in a safe and hygienic environment.

c) Prevent the diversion of prescribed heroin to the illicit market.

Clients could come to the clinics up to three times a day, get their injections, wait for twenty minutes and go back. These clinics were located in densely populated areas so commuting time was minimal. Thus, stigma and isolation were reduced by sending a message that this was just another treatment.

This was a sign of acceptance by society of the simple but uncomfortable fact that a good number of patients keep having craving for heroin even while on Methadone or Buprenorphine and relapse frequently. And that as a last option, society might as well give them heroin in clinics under supervision so that they spend less time in trying to acquire the drug, thus letting them spend that time at work and with family and friends, reducing markedly the number of overdosage deaths and HIV and Hepatitis infections. Since heroin here was being used for treatment under medical supervision it bypassed the prohibitions under the UN conventions.

Most patients, rather than asking for a higher and higher dose after an initial phase of insecurity, stabilized it themselves and then slowly reduced the dose overtime, thus proving that given autonomy, persons with addiction do act responsibly as long as there is the security of availability. Giving control to the persons themselves was enabling and empowered the patients to reduce and taper off. As they had more time and more mind space to work and socialise instead of worrying about where to get the next supply from, they began to integrate into society better. At the end of three years, only 15% were still taking heroin. Others had tapered it off on their own.

There was an immediate fall in the crime rate earlier associated with acquisition of drugs illegally at extortionate prices. Muggings were down by 80%. This also brought the addicts out of the criminal ecosystem.

In 1985, 68% of all AIDS patients in Switzerland were injectable heroin addicts. In 2009, this was down to 5%, substantially decreasing the country's public health expense. A third of the addicts who had been on welfare came off it as they became independent. The number of addicts dying of AIDS went down dramatically and the proportion of persons with permanent jobs tripled in the long run.

The programme costs thirty-five Swiss Francs per patient

per day and it saves the government forty-four Francs per day per user, which was earlier spent on arresting, trying and jailing them. This was in addition to massive savings in the public health expenditure earlier incurred on the management of the drug-related AIDS epidemic. In 2008, the right-wing Swiss People's Party organized a national referendum on heroin-assisted treatment. A clear majority of people (68%) voted in favour of continuing the Swiss HAT Programme.

After the success of the Swiss HAT Programme, Canada, Germany, the Netherlands, Spain and the United Kingdom have embarked on the experimental implementation of such initiatives over the past decades.

A detailed review of the studies done on all the initiatives in these countries was published in 2007 in the *Journal of Urban Health*. It was titled, 'Heroin-assisted Treatment a Decade Later: A Brief Update on Science and Politics'. The review concluded, 'the discussed studies have demonstrated in several different contexts that the implementation of HAT is feasible, effective and safe as a therapeutic intervention.' This should not be seen as a conclusion that could be taken for granted because many observers expected the bold experiment to have disastrous consequences.

Uruguay: the tiny South American country wedged between Argentina and Brazil, has made possession of *small quantities of all drugs for personal use legal* like Portugal. Production and sale, however, remain illegal as before, again as in Portugal. No threshold quantities are laid down and the courts decide the doubtful cases on a case-to-case basis whether the drug in a person's possession is for commercial or personal use.

More radically, in 2014, Uruguay also became the first country in Latin America to legalise cannabis for recreational use. Since 2017, cannabis sale has been legal though regulated like alcohol in India, but with stricter controls. Customers have to register with the regulator and then are limited to buying 10 gms a week, enough for about twenty joints. The regulator also controls how strong the marijuana is. The level of THC is balanced with the level of CBD, another compound in the plant that is said to have a calming effect. Since marijuana went on sale, the novelty of the experiment may have waned, but the queues have not.

Guillermo Draper, a Uruguayan journalist who has co-written a book on his country's bold and successful experiment said it took time because they wanted to do it step by step. The expenditure on prosecuting and jailing people has come down and the only people troubled by the reform seem to be the US banks, which are in partnership with Uruguayan banks. They have pressurized their local partners to not finance 'cannabis pharmacies' as the stores which sell cannabis for recreational use are called.

'My bank told me to either stop selling cannabis or close my accounts,' says Esteban Riviera, a pharmacist. 'I stopped selling cannabis...Mine was the first pharmacy registered to sell cannabis, but it was also the first that stopped selling cannabis in Uruguay.'

The USA: While American banks were busy arm twisting their Uruguayan partners into withdrawing funding from local stores selling weed legally, twenty-one states and District of Columbia in the USA legalized the recreational use of cannabis. This despite the fact that US federal law continues to treat the possession of cannabis for personal use a crime, reflecting a schizophrenia of sorts in the minds of American policy makers. As many as thirty-six US states have legalized marijuana for medical use, including treatment of chronic pain. In what seems to be a highly promising scenario, in a report published in the Journal of the American Medical Association in 2018, the authors reported that availability of cannabis was associated with significant reductions in opioid prescriptions for chronic pain in the states where cannabis was allowed for medical or recreational use. Prescription opioids are at present a significant contributor to the overall opioid crisis in the USA including high overdosage deaths.

Satisfied with their experiment of legalising the recreational use of cannabis in 2015, the state of Oregon went ahead and *decriminalized all drugs* including heroin, meth and cocaine in November 2020. In a landmark vote, Oregon voters approved 'Measure 110', which decriminalizes all drugs including heroin, cocaine and methamphetamine. Thus, *Oregon became the first US state to decriminalize possession and personal use of all drugs.* CNN (Nov 9, 2020) reported, 'The initiative also expands access to addiction assistance and other health services, offering aid to those who need it instead of arresting and jailing people for drugs. Possession of drugs such as heroin, cocaine and methamphetamine will no longer be punishable by jail time, but instead amount to something similar to a traffic ticket. Measure 110 is arguably the biggest blow to date to the War on Drugs. It shifts the focus to where it belongs–on people and public health–and removes one of the most common justifications for law enforcement to harass, arrest, prosecute, incarcerate and deport people.'

In the USA, a grim milestone was crossed when overdose deaths rose to more than 100,000 in the twelve-month period that ended in April 2021, according to the National Centre for Health Statistics, up nearly 30% from the previous twelve months. More than 2,000 people died of a drug overdose in

New York City in 2020, the highest total since the city began keeping track of overdose deaths in 2000. During the first three months of 2021, there were close to 600 overdose deaths according to preliminary data.

As a calculated harm reduction measure, New York city opened the nation's first two supervized drug-injection sites, 'facilities that opponents view as magnets for drug abuse but proponents praise as providing a less punitive and more effective approach to addressing addiction' (*The New York Times*, November 30, 2021).

Trained staff at two sites—in the neighbourhoods of East Harlem and Washington Heights—provided clean needles, administered Naloxone to reverse overdoses and provided users with options for addiction treatment. Users brought their own drugs to the sites. In an interview, Dr Dave A. Chokshi, the city's health commissioner, said New York was moving forward to address a public health crisis. 'Every four hours, someone dies of a drug overdose in New York City,' he said. 'We feel a deep conviction and also a sense of urgency in opening overdose prevention centres.' On the first day, the trained staff reversed two overdosage cases, persons who would have otherwise died at home.

Other cities including Philadelphia, San Francisco, Boston and Seattle have taken steps towards supervized injection, but have yet to open sites amidst a raging debate over the legal and moral implications of sanctioning illegal drug and humane and scientific harm reduction measures. A study from California published in March 2021 reported that supervized injection sites actually decreased rather than increased the crime rate in the community over five years and that concerns about safe consumption sites attracting crime were unwarranted.

Other countries: Canada, South Africa, Georgia and some parts of Australia have also liberalized the recreational use of cannabis. In addition, the Netherlands has long had a tolerant cannabis policy, which allows the recreational use and limited sale of cannabis by the authorities looking the other way.

Some early reports have shown that in Canada, after cannabis was legalized, beer sales have shown some decrease. In the states where the recreational use of cannabis is now legal, binge drinking in students is less than in the states where recreational use continues to be illegal. Financial experts estimate that newly legal pot products like vapes, edibles and cannabis beverages will further perpetuate this trend of declining beer volumes. In an interesting study by David Kerr and colleagues published in the journal, *Addiction* (2017), it is noted that the rates of Oregon college students' marijuana use increased (relative to that of students in other states) following the recreational marijuana legislation in 2015, but only among those who reported recent heavy use of alcohol. This fits in with the case for making milder intoxicants more available. When you liberalise the availability of a milder intoxicant, chances are that over a period of time, it will partly replace a harder intoxicant as the preferred choice.

~

Before we focus on the possibility of liberalising drugs in India, let us remind ourselves once more about what happens when a drug is decriminalised or legalized. When a drug is decriminalised, it is no longer a crime to use it but it is still a crime to sell it. The fact is that some more people will use it at least initially. But this would likely be a small increase because one still has to access illegal sellers who operate in shady places. Once a drug is legalized it becomes lawfully available to adults in regulated stores just like alcohol. Whenever somebody advocates legalization, the impression many people get is that what is being advocated is a 'smoke, swallow, inject or inhale whatever you feel like' i.e., a free for all scenario. However, this is a misconception. Most advocates of legalization want drugs to be made available only to adults in government approved licensed stores like in Canada, Uruguay and twenty-one states in the USA.

While legalization will increase the number of users to an extent, many will be first time users or experimental users. After their first try, many will not like the experience and may not use a drug ever again. But they will be counted as users if a survey is done the following year. The National Magnitude Survey counted all those who had in the previous year drank a beer, inhaled a whiff or consumed a sleeping tablet as users. Generally, when we talk of users, we are referring to people who take a drug casually and periodically. We are not talking of persons who are addicted.

Consider the example of cannabis. There are some people who do not even think of smoking weed because it is illegal. A law is a law and they follow it. If they feel like getting slightly intoxicated on a weekend, they will stick to having a beer or two. What if weed becomes available in stores like liquor? Some of them will shift from alcohol to weed and this will lead to an increase in the number of cannabis users. However, if we are convinced that casual use of weed is not more harmful than casual use of alcohol, we can easily live with the increased numbers of cannabis users because those numbers would have come from the population of alcohol users. Similarly, some users of heroin or other synthetic opioids who are tired of the immense risks involved in getting their hands on the drugs will shift to smoking weed.

Again, we can live with that because it is even easier to

understand that the casual use of cannabis is potentially much less harmful than the casual use of synthetic opioids like heroin. The logical assumption here is that all drugs are harmful and if people have to use a drug, any measure which makes them use less harmful drugs should be considered as a serious option by society.

In the Netherlands, after cannabis was liberalized in 1976, there was no increase in its user base. However, seven years later, the Netherlands legalized it and allowed licensed cafes to sell cannabis (although this is not officially called legalization for the fear of offending the UN and the USA). After it was made legally available, there was an increase in the number of persons using cannabis. Part of this increase was also because of the fact that when a drug is made legal, more people are likely to admit to having used it than when it was illegal. The important point to note is that things did not slip out of control in the Netherlands after cannabis was legalized. And the country still has lesser rates of cannabis use than other European countries where cannabis sale and use are criminal offences.

The other serious concern about the legalization of any drug is that more minors will use it if it is available legally. Three years back, I found myself in the quaintly beautiful city of Portland, USA. After a long evening walk along a forest trail, I sighted a bar and decided to have a beer. I had to wait for ten minutes in a queue because it was Friday evening and the man at the door was taking his own time checking photo-ids for age proof, before letting customers in. Although I clearly looked much older than twenty-one, the legal age of drinking in Oregon, my proof of age was diligently verified.

When I walked out an hour later, I saw a man seated inside a car parked in a dark corner of the parking lot selling drugs to a group of youngsters, a couple of whom were clearly minors.

And I thought to myself, suppose whatever drug the man was selling was legal, it would at least not be sold to kids because while legal entities check age proof, smugglers do not. Many years ago, a study involving American teenagers found that a large number of teens found it easier to buy weed than alcohol.

If we legalise a drug, the age check would be a barrier between that drug and minors, a barrier which does not exist at present.

The third, and equally serious concern is that if more people take a drug, proportionately more will eventually end up being addicted to it. However, this relation between availability, use and addiction seems to be true only up to a limited point. Cigarettes continue to be available freely, but the incidence of tobacco addiction through smoking has come down by about half all over the world. This is because people's awareness of the harmful effects of tobacco has increased. Just because a product known to be harmful is legal and freely available does not mean that people flock in large numbers to use it. Alcohol is available freely in India but 85.4% of Indians are teetotallers.

In Portugal, when all drugs were liberalized, the usage increased but addiction actually decreased because the youngsters who were previously caught up in the rigmarole of arrests, bail, prison, parole, etc., because of their drug use were now free to take charge of their lives. Because of the absence of stigma and the hassle-free, long stretches of time now made available to them, they could get on with jobs and to reconnecting with society in emotionally enriching ways.

~

Both the Portugal and Switzerland experiments, which are considered remarkable successes by scientists today were essentially bold initiatives undertaken by politicians who had observed for years the misery caused by the War on Drugs from close quarters. They understood the fact that drugs are not going anywhere even if ten such wars were waged. They asked wisely, 'Can we significantly decrease the harms caused by drugs without necessarily trying to eradicate them altogether?' They trusted their experts and believed in the science of the day. Most significantly, they favoured pragmatic outcomes based on logic rather than ideal but illogical outcomes based on sentimental morality. Will policy makers in India, especially in states like Punjab, be able to take such radical and scientifically sound reforms if experts propose they do so?

There are a few crucial voices out there, who can provide the blueprint for future drug reforms in India. Dr Dharamveer Gandhi is a popular physician in Patiala. Up to 2019, he was a member of Parliament. During his stint as a Lok Sabha member, he piloted a private members' bill in 2017, proposing the decriminalization of use and possession of small quantities of drugs, access to natural opiates to those addicted and allowing farmers to grow cannabis for medical and industrial use. He pointed out that people in Punjab have been consuming opium and other natural intoxicants for centuries and there have been no recorded fatalities because of this. The bill however could not be discussed since a large number of private members' bill are always pending and are taken up for discussion by a draw of lots and Dr Gandhi's bill was not lucky.

Dr Gandhi works for twelve hours a day, six days of the week. He is a poor man's cardiologist, seeing over a hundred patients a day and charging a hundred rupees as consultation fees from those who can afford it. For the poor, everything is free including medicines. I met him on a Sunday morning in his spacious yet simple clinic. He was dressed in a pyjama, a shirt and a modest shawl. The Lenin bust on the mantelpiece completed the austere picture. Dr Gandhi was born and brought up in a village in what is now Ropar district bordering Himachal Pradesh. He talked about his childhood days in the village when there was just one liquor vend for a hundred villages. Opium husk and opium were used but sparingly except during the back-breaking harvest months when farm hands were handed poppy husk, which they took every day during those months. But drug addiction was never a problem.

Opium and natural products of opium did not make the persons dysfunctional or rowdy. According to Dr Gandhi, opium and its husk were called *'kamaau nasha'* and *'saau nasha,'* meaning, the people who used these continued to be productive, gentle and well-behaved members of Punjabi society. 'Before 1985, drugs never killed anybody,' he said. 'Nor did they wreck Punjabi society.'

He added, 'Drugs did not damage Punjab. NDPS did. And now that terrorism has died down, the politicians and the police have latched on to NDPS as a money-making machine. Half the large properties in Mohali are bought with money extorted out of NDPS victims. They are heavily invested in NDPS and want it to continue.'

There are many people in Punjab who agree with him and advocate a liberalization of substances. Some even go on to suggest that cannabis and hemp cultivation may be the much-needed diversifications required from the rote wheat-paddy cycle. That such conversations are happening at all is cause for hope.

The NDPS Act was amended in 2001 to allow more scientific drug research and encourage private industry to enter the international pharmaceutical opium market. Uttarakhand recently became the first state in India to legalize the production of industrial cannabis. These steps at least symbolically carry a hope of salvation from the problem of complete prohibition, which continues to ensnare some other Indian states.

Whenever an argument is made in support of the liberalization of cannabis, one of the counter-arguments that comes up is about its role in causing acute psychotic episodes. This is indeed a valid argument, and it would be irresponsible not to address this issue particularly when we are talking about young and vulnerable people. Several studies over the last seven decades have shown that cannabis does indeed increase the chances of psychotic episodes in those who take it. The latest is a vast multicentred study conducted all over Europe by Forti et al titled, 'The contribution of cannabis use to variation in the incidence of psychotic disorder across Europe.' It was reported in the March 2019 issue of *The Lancet*.

The study found that among the cases of first-time acute psychotic episodes, 64% had a history of cannabis use in the past while in the age-matched normal controls, 46% had such a history. Far more importantly, psychotic episodes occurred more frequently in the cohort, which took high potency cannabis products of above 10% THC content or took cannabis every day. Only legalization and regulated sale can ensure that adults are issued a fixed amount of a standard marijuana product below a particular level of THC content. Peddlers and smugglers have no such commitment to society. *Cannabis and other drugs should be legalized not because these are safe but because these are not. Regulation will make these safer.*

At the heart of the liberalization debate is the fact that all addictions are harmful but some addictions are far more harmful than others. The goal here is not the romantic ideal of harm eradication, because that has proven to be impossible. A more pragmatic harm reduction is the goal.

Another argument commonly voiced against legalization of

cannabis is that even if it is presumed that it is not so harmful in itself, it may act as a gateway drug and it may be used as a stepping stone to harder drugs like cocaine or heroin. However, the gateway theory popular in the seventies and eighties suffers from many methodological flaws. At present, it is unable to specify a one-to-one causal relationship between early use of any specific drug and the potential to use or abuse other drugs later. Instead, these relationships may be more consistent with the common liability model according to which the vulnerability to addiction is generic and using nearly any drug early on is associated with a higher potential to abuse other drugs later. By this model of common liability, any drug could be a 'gateway drug' for any other drug in the case of persons who have a general propensity to develop addiction because of genetic and experiential factors.

~

Even if we leave other countries aside and focus only on what India has achieved by waging the exorbitant War on Drugs since we promulgated the NDPS Act in 1985, there is absolutely nothing to console ourselves with. This War has been costly not just in terms of the money spent on policing, prosecuting and jailing people but even more importantly, in terms of its human cost. Thousands of young men, most of whom are peddlers and users caught with small quantities of drugs, are in jail. And what is the gain reaped from it?

The number of persons with addiction to hard and dangerous drugs has increased astronomically. The number of persons suffering from potentially fatal diseases like AIDS and Hepatitis-C acquired through injecting drugs are several times more than what it was before 1985. On the treatment front, we are woefully short of manpower and infrastructural and technical resources because of increasing numbers. Whatever resources we have, we cannot use them optimally because of the existing stigma and morality-based prejudices against persons with addiction in the minds of policy makers, administrators and even doctors working for the administration.

Whenever we ask such questions of ourselves and others, we are told that seizure of illegal drugs has been exponentially increasing over the years. This is true but what does it mean for the future when all other indicators are becoming worse every year? During the year 2019, 3,000 kgs of heroin and 4,400 kgs of opium were seized by India's drug enforcement agencies. This is a very impressive haul but as Dr Atul Ambekar of the National Drug Dependence Treatment Centre put it in perspective, this is just 5-8% of the heroin and opium consumed in one year by persons with opium/heroin dependence in India (*The Times of India*, November 9, 2020).

If we follow this line of thinking, we will need to put in twenty times more effort, personnel and money just to catch up with stopping the current supply of heroin, and of course by then the numbers would have galloped ahead. Many other countries in the world have realized this and stepped back from the purely coercive law and order approach. As Dr Ambekar stressed, the focus has to be on simultaneously decreasing the demand not just the supply. And demand can be decreased only by having more and better treatment facilities and by increasing awareness. The demand for strong and harmful drugs like heroin can be decreased by legalising and regulating milder drugs like cannabis and plant-based opioids.

The question should not be how to rid society of all drugs because as history as well as recent experience tells us this is impossible for many reasons. Most importantly, the roots of drug use and addiction cannot be eradicated because those roots lie in the human brain. The question should be how to minimise the devastation caused by addictions to individuals and societies.

Here is a set of recommendations formulated in the light of the aspects and observations that have been discussed in detail in this book:

1. We should decriminalise the use and possession of small quantities of all currently illicit drugs like the Netherlands, Portugal, Uruguay and Oregon in the US have done. These individuals need treatment and not incarceration. Since most people arrested and jailed in India at the moment are users and petty peddlers, it will drastically reduce the public expenditure of hundreds of billions of rupees spent by the government in arresting and jailing such people.

2. We should regulate and make available a certain THC content cannabis preparation like bhang and marijuana in fixed amounts from government approved outlets to adults for recreational use, just like alcohol is at present.

This is already being done in the Netherlands, twenty-one states of the USA, Argentina, Uruguay, Canada, Spain, Switzerland, the Czech Republic and parts of Australia.

3. Mild plant-based opiates like poppy husk should be legalized along the same lines as proposed by Dr Gandhi in his bill before parliament. Initially, the Northeastern and the Northwestern states may be chosen to start this process where injectable heroin intake, overdosage deaths, HIV and Hepatitis-C infections are high.

An argument can be made that unscrupulous elements might buy these drugs from government approved outlets and hoard and sell these illegally. However, if it does not happen to alcohol, why would it happen to cannabis and poppy husk? And why would anyone buy these drugs in the black market and risk jail when these are available legally in stores? Additionally, the government will receive a large amount of revenue as taxes which can be used for prevention, treatment and rehabilitation of persons with addiction.

4. Persons using drugs in public, individually or in groups, should be mandatorily referred to social workers and psychologists for counselling for safe use of drugs and assessment. If found to be addicted or involved in the harmful use of drugs, they should be referred for treatment which should be voluntary, confidential and either cheap or free.

5. Drugs awareness programmes should be an essential part of the school curriculum and should be run by the students themselves so that youngsters can talk freely about their individual views.

6. The country should have a syringes/needles programme to reach out to all communities in order to deal with the rising numbers of persons infected and dying from HIV and Hepatitis-C.

7. For persons addicted to opioid drugs, who need treatment counselling and oral substitution treatment, programmes should be expanded all over the country to include carry home medications, both Buprenorphine and Methadone. The government should subsidise these programmes for those who cannot pay.

8. We should form an expert committee to look into the possible use of medically pure heroin under medical supervision in government clinics for patients for whom all other treatments have failed. We should recognise the fact there will always be a group of patients who will continue to have craving on conventional OST medications. The larger purpose here would be to decrease the number of overdosage deaths and bring under control the very high number of persons infected with Hepatitis-C and HIV as a result of shared needles.

~

Addiction is a chronic disease like hypertension, diabetes or rheumatoid arthritis, which can be managed like these illnesses but cannot be eradicated. However, out of the myriad forms of addiction, some are much more harmful to individuals and to society than others. In addition to managing addictions, efforts can be made to replace devastating addictions like heroin addiction with much less harmful ones. The only choice available is about how much of which addiction a society wants to have at a particular time and that choice is relative at best. From this perspective, it makes sense to liberalize milder intoxicants. The war against drugs has gone on for far too long at an enormous cost to humanity. It is time to make peace.

References

CHAPTER 1

Inglis, Lucy. 2018. *Milk of Paradise: A History of Opium*. Pan Macmillan.

Nath, Dwarka. 1965. United Nations Office on Drugs and Crime. https://www.unodc.org/unodc/en/data-and-analysis/bulletin/bulletin_1965-01-01_1_page004.html1 (last accessed September 5, 2021).

'Some Temples in North Karnataka Give Marijuana as Prasada'. *The Times of India,* September 7, 2020.

https://timesofindia.indiatimes.com/city/hubballi/some-temples-in-north-karnataka-give-marijuana-as-prasada/articleshow/77969163.cms (last accessed on December 15, 2021).

Kapur, R. K. 1931. 'A History of the Excise System in the Punjab'. Punjab Government Record Office, Lahore.

Chardin, John. 2003. *Travels in Persia*, 1673-77. Dover Publications Inc.

Toussaint, Eric. 2014. 'HSBC: the bank with a shameful past and scandalous present', Committee for Abolition of Illegitimate Debt, https://www.cadtm.org/HSBC-the-bank-with-a-shameful-past (last accessed on September 5, 2021).

The Report of the Royal Commission on Opium (1895). *British Medical Journal.* April 13, 1895; 1(1789): 836-37. https://www.ncbi.nlm.nih.gov/pmc/articles/PMC2509215/ (last accessed on September 5, 2021).

Jehangir, Rustom Pestonji. 2019. *A Short History of the Lives of Bombay Opium Smokers*. Wentworth Press.

Chopra, Ram Nath and Chopra I. C. 1955. 'Quasi-medical Use of Opium in India and its Effects', United Nations Office on Drug and Crime. https://www.unodc.org/unodc/en/data-and-analysis/bulletin/bulletin_1955-01-01_3_page002.html (last accessed on September 7, 2021).

The Indian Hemp Drugs Commission, 1893–94. (May, 2019) https://www.researchgate.net/publication/332886341_The_Indian_Hemp_Drugs_Commission_1893-1894 (last accessed on September 7, 2021).

United Nations Office on Drugs and Crime (2018) https://www.unodc.org/wdr2018/prelaunch/WDR18_Booklet_3_DRUG_MARKETS.pdf. (last accessed on September 7, 2021).

'Narco-Jihad–Haram Money for a Halal cause?' (2017). European Society for South Asian Studies. https://www.efsas.org/publications/study-papers/%E2%80%98narco-jihad%E2%80%99-%E2%80%93-haram-money-for-a-halal-cause/ (last accessed September 7, 2021).

UNODC Reports Major, and Growing, Drug Abuse in Afghanistan (2010). https://www.unodc.org/unodc/en/press/releases/2010/June/unodc-reports-major-and-growing-drug-abuse-in-afghanistan.html (last accessed on September 7, 2021).

Chopra, Ram Nath. 'The Present Position of the Opium Habit in India'. 1928. *Indian Journal of Medical Research*, Issue: 16.

Booth, Martin. 2003. *Cannabis*. Bantam Books.

CHAPTER 2

Kapur R. K. 1931. 'A History of the Excise system in the Punjab'. Punjab Government Record Office, Lahore.

'Alcohol consumption patterns in India'. 2021. *Ambrosia*, the Magazine for the alcohol industry. https://www.ambrosiaindia.com/2021/02/4494/ (last accessed on September 8, 2021).

Singh, Dalbir. 'Rise, Growth and Fall of Bhangi Misal'. PhD

(2010) thesis submitted to the Department of History, Punjab University.) http://citeseerx.ist.psu.edu/viewdoc/download?doi=10.1.1.693.6648&rep=rep1&type=pdf. (last accessed on September 12, 2021).

Ambekar A, Agrawal A, Rao R, Mishra A. K., Khandelwal S.K. and Chadda R.K. on behalf of the group of investigators for the National Survey on Extent and Pattern of Substance Use in India (2019). Magnitude of Substance Use in India, 2019. New Delhi: Ministry of Social Justice and Empowerment, Government of India.

Sachdev, Jaswant Singh; Yakhmi, Ranvir Singh and Sharma, Ajay Kumar. 2002. 'Changing Pattern of Drug Abuse Among Patients Attending De-addiction Centre at Faridkot'. *Indian Journal of Psychiatry.* 44 (4). 353-55.

Single Convention on Narcotic Drugs, 1961. As amended by the 1972 Protocol. https://www.unodc.org/pdf/convention_1961_en.pdf (last accessed on September 12, 2021).

'Punjab earns Rs 8.8 lakh from cannabis sale'. *The Times of India*, May 13, 2014.

https://timesofindia.indiatimes.com/india/punjab-earns-rs-8-8-lakh-from-cannabis-sale/articleshow/35040705.cms (last accessed on September 12, 2021).

CHAPTER 3

The Indian Express, January 13, 2020. https://indianexpress.com/article/cities/ chandigarh/in-four-years- punjab-rejected-61-1-farm-suicide- cases -as-ineligible-6214530/ (last accessed on September 13, 2021).

Howe Colt, George. 1991. *The Enigma of Suicide.* Simon and Schuster.com https://books.google.co.in/books?id=DOz3hStePfYC&pg=PA201&lpg=PA201&dq=karl+meninger+partial+suicides&source=bl&ots=Ew_fRmZJWR&sig=ACfU3U1pYHj2LDhBx192NADn3LO0mZxaFw&hl=en&sa=X&ved=2ahUKEwid2J7Bp

PnyAhUr6nMBHd0jAugQ6AF6BAgTEAM#v=onepage&q=
karl%20meninger%20partial%20suicides&f=false (last accessed
on September 13, 2021).

Dunlap, Eloise; Golub, Andrew and D. Johnson, Bruce. 2006. 'The
Severely-Distressed African American Family in the Crack Era:
Empowerment is not Enough'. *Journal of Social Soc Welfare.*
33 (1): 115-139. https://www.ncbi.nlm.nih.gov/pmc/ articles/
PMC2565489/ (last accessed on September 13, 2021).

Alexander B.K.; Beyerstein B.L.; Hadaway B.F. and Coombs R.B. 1981.
'Effect of Early and Later Colony Housing on Oral Ingestion of
Morphine in Rats'. *Pharmacol Biochem Behav.* 15: 571-76.

Chauvet, Claudia et al. 2009. 'Environmental Enrichment Reduces
Cocaine Seeking and Reinstatement Induced by Cues and
Stress but Not by Cocaine'. *Neuropsychopharmacology.* 34 (13):
2767-2778. doi:10.1038/npp.2009.127. PMC 3178884. PMID
19741591.

Solinas et al. April 2009. 'Reversal of cocaine addiction by
environmental enrichment'. *Neuropsychopharmacology.* 34 (5):
1102-11. doi:10.1038/npp.2008.51. PMC 2579392. PMID
18955698.

CHAPTER 4

Hari, John. 2019. *Chasing the Scream: The Search for the Truth About
Addiction.* Bloomsbury Publishing, UK.

Vidhi Legal Report. Volumes I & II. 'From Addict to Convict, The
Working of the NDPS Act (1985) in Punjab'. Vidhi Centre for
Legal Policy, New Delhi, 2018.

Lawyers' Collective. 2018. A critical look at Vidhi Centre's 'From
Addict to Convict: Working of the NDPS Act in Punjab' Report.
https://theleaflet.in/wp-content/uploads/2018/09/Critique-
Vidhi-Addict-to-Convict-Report-2018-.pdf (last accessed on
September 15, 2021).

National Crime Records Bureau (2020). Crime in India, 2020.
https://ncrb.gov.in/en/Crime-in-India-2020 (last accessed on
September 16, 2021).

War on Drugs: Report of the Global Commission on Drug Policy (2011). https://www.opensociety foundations.org/publications/war-drugs-report-global-commission-drug-policy (last accessed on September 17, 2021).

Singhal, Neha. 'Narcotics Law: It's Not Just About Celebrities.' *The Times of India,* October 29, 2021.

CHAPTER 5

Courtwright, David T. 2002. *Forces of Habit: Drugs and the Making of the Modern World.* 2022. Harvard University Press.

'Reducing Risks and Promoting Health Lives', WHO. 2002. http://apps.who.int/iris/bitstream/handle/10665/67454/WHO_WHR_02.1.pdf;jsessionid=5E6DE9F4F0540163B78DF5BC777729AF?sequence=1 (last accessed on September 24, 2021).

Magnitude of Substance Use in India, 2019. Ministry of Social Justice & Empowerment and National Drug Dependence & Treatment Centre, All India Institute of Medical Sciences, New Delhi.

http://www.ndusindia.in/report.html (last accessed on September 12, 2021).

Alcohol Use and Burden for 195 Countries and Territories, 1990-2016: A Systematic Analysis for the Global Burden of Disease Study 2016. GBD Alcohol Collaborators. *The Lancet,* 2018. https://www.thelancet.com/article/S0140-6736(18)31310-2/fulltext (last accessed on September 25, 2021).

National Family Health Survey, 2019-21

https://timesofindia.indiatimes.com/india/fewer-indians-are-drinking-but-some-are-drinking-harder/articleshow/91658145.cms (last accessed on May 23, 2022).

Population-level Risks of Alcohol Consumption by Amount, Geography, Age, Sex and Year: A Systematic Analysis for the Global Burden of Disease Study 2020. GBD 2020 Alcohol Collaborators. *The Lancet,* Vol. 400. No. 10347. 137-250. July 16, 2022. https://www.thelancet.com/journals/lancet/issue/vol400no10347/PIIS0140-6736(22)X0029-9 retrieved July 18, 2022.

CHAPTER 6

Magnitude of Substance Use in India, 2019. Ministry of Social Justice & Empowerment and National Drug Dependence & Treatment Centre, All India Institute of Medical Sciences, New Delhi. http://www.ndusindia.in/report.html (last accessed on September 12, 2021).

Global Status Report on Alcohol and Health. 2018. WHO. https://www.who.int/publications/i/item/ 9789241565639 (last accessed on September 29, 2021).

Global Adult Tobacco Survey Fact Sheet | India 2016-17. World Health Organization. https://www.who.int/tobacco/surveillance/survey/gats/ GATS_India_2016-17_FactSheet.pdf (last accessed on September 29, 2021).

National Survey on Extent, Pattern and Trends of Drug Abuse in India, 2004. United Nations Office on Drugs & Crime. https://www.unodc.org/pdf/india/presentations/india_national_survey_2004.pdf (last accessed on September 29, 2021).

'In Two Years, only 70 Register at Government Rehab Centre for Women'. *The Tribune.* https://www.tribuneindia.com/news/punjab/in-2-years-only-70-register-at-govt-rehab-centre-for-women/782125.html (last accessed on September 29, 2021).

CHAPTER 7

National Institute on Drug Abuse, 2021, Overdose Death Rates. https://www.drugabuse.gov/drug-topics/trends-statistics/overdose-death-rates (last accessed on October 1, 2021).

Opioid Overdose (2021). WHO. https://www.who.int/news-room/fact-sheets/detail/opioid-overdose (last accessed on October 1, 2021).

CHAPTER 8

Siegel, Ronald K. 2005. *Intoxication: The Universal Drive for Mind-Altering Substances.* Park Street Press.

Drug Use in Pakistan, 2013. United Nations Office on Drugs and Crime https://www.unodc.org/unodc/en/frontpage/2013/March/Key-findings-of-the-drug-use-in-pakistan-2013-technical-summary- report.html (last accessed on October 2, 2021).

Magnitude of Substance Use in India, 2019. Ministry of Social Justice & Empowerment and National Drug Dependence & Treatment Centre, All India Institute of Medical Sciences, New Delhi.

Dodes L. 2002. *The Heart of Addiction*. New York: HarperCollins.

CHAPTER 9

Maté, Gabe. 2010. *In the Realm of Hungry Ghosts: Close Encounters with Addiction*. North Atlantic Books.

Yale Food Addiction Scale. Gearhardt, Ashley N., R. Corbin, William and D. Brownell, Kelly (YFAS). https://www.midss.org/content/yale-food-addiction-scale-yfas (last accessed October 19, 2021).

CHAPTER 10

Tobacco, Alcohol and Drug Use in Eight to Sixteen-year-old Twins: The Virginia Twin Study of Adolescent Behavioral Development, H. H. Maes I; C. E. Woodard; L. Murrelle; J. M. Meyer; J. L. Silberg; J. K. Hewitt; M. Rutter; E. Simonoff; A. Pickles; R. Carbonneau; M. C. Neale and L. J. Eaves. 1999. https://pubmed.ncbi.nlm.nih.gov/10371255/ (last accessed on October 4, 2021).

Tonmyr, Lil and Shields, Margot. 2016. 'Childhood Sexual Abuse and Substance Abuse: A Gender Paradox?' https://www.sciencedirect.com/science/ article/pii/S0145213416302551 (last accessed on October 4, 2021).

F.S. Cohen and J. Densen-Gerber. 1982. A study of the relationship between child abuse and drug addiction in 178 patients: preliminary results. https://pubmed.ncbi.nlm.nih.gov/6892324/ (last accessed on October 4, 2021).

Mukherjee, Bhaskar. 2019. Personal communication.

Maté, Gabe. 2010. *In the Realm of Hungry Ghosts: Close Encounters with Addiction*. North Atlantic Books.

CHAPTER 11 AND 12

Holiday, Billie. 1915-59. https://www.biography.com/musician/billie-holiday (last accessed on October 6, 2021).

Methadone and Buprenorphine added to the WHO list of essential medicines. https://pubmed.ncbi.nlm.nih.gov/16544403/ (last accessed on October 6, 2021).

'Hooked on De-addiction Pill. Haryana Youth, Too, Falling in Buprenorphine Trap.' *The Tribune,* Chandigarh, June 28, 2022. https://www.tribuneindia.com/news/editorials/hooked-on-de-addiction-pill-407195 (last accessed on June 28, 2022).

'Only 0.5% of Drug Users Get Medical Care'. Hindu.com, September 26, 2019 https://www.thehindu.com/news/cities/Kochi/only-05-of-drug-users-get-medical-care/article29513411.ece (last accessed on January 2, 2023).

Punjab Police Tweets, "#DrugAddiction reduces a man to a mindless and ridiculous thing, and creates social parasites and criminals. #SayNotoDrugs.' https://twitter.com/PunjabPoliceInd/status/ 1585821237195853825

CHAPTER 13

A Brief History of the Drug War. Drug Policy Alliance, 2021. https://drugpolicy.org/issues/brief-history-drug-war (last accessed on October 15, 2021).

'Global patterns of opioid use and dependence: harms to populations, interventions, and future action'. *The Lancet.* October 2019. 394 (10208).

Miron, Jeffrey A. 2010. 'The Budgetary Implications of Drug Prohibition'. Cambridge: Department of Economics; 1-39.

Miron, Jeffrey A. 2004. 'Drug War Crimes: The Consequences of Prohibition'. Oakland, California.

United Nations Convention Against Illicit Traffic in Narcotic Drugs and Psychotropics Substances, 1988. https://www.unodc.org/pdf/convention_1988_en.pdf (last accessed on October 16, 2021).

Hari, John. 2019. *Chasing the Scream: The Search for the Truth About Addiction.* Bloomsbury Publishing, UK.

Drug Decriminalization in Portugal: Lessons for Creating Fair and Successful Drug Policies. April 2, 2009. White Paper. https://www.cato.org/white-paper/drug-decriminalization-portugal-lessons-creating-fair-successful-drug- policies (last accessed on October 16, 2021).

Drug Decriminalization in Portugal: Challenges and Limitations, The White House, 2009. https://obamawhitehouse.archives.gov/ondcp/ondcp-fact-sheets/drug-decriminalization-in-portugal-challenges-and- limitations (last accessed on October 16, 2021).

Fischer, B.; Oviedo-Joekes, E.; Blanken, P. et al. 'Heroin-assisted Treatment (HAT) a Decade Later: A Brief Update on Science and Politics'. 2007. *Journal of Urban Health.* 84, 552-62.

'Oregon Measure Decriminalising Small Amounts of Drugs Takes Effect in a First in US'. February 2, 2021. https://www.nbcnews.com/news/ us-news/oregon-measure-decriminalizing-possession-drugs-takes-effect- first-u-s-n1256436 (last accessed on October 16, 2021).

Kerr D.C. R.; Bae H.; Phibbs S. and Kern A.C. November 2017. 'Changes in undergraduates' marijuana, heavy alcohol and cigarette use following legalization of recreational marijuana use in Oregon'. *Addiction.* 112 (11) :1992-2001. doi: 10.1111/add.13906. Epub 2017 Jul 11. PMID: 28613454.

The Contribution of Cannabis Use to Variation in the Incidence of Psychotic Disorder across Europe (EU-GEI): A Multicentre Case-control Study. *The Lancet Psychiatry*, Vol. 6, Issue 5, 427-36. May 1, 2019. Di Forti, Marta, PhD; Quattrone, Diego, MD; P. Freeman, Tom, PhD; Tripoli, Giada, MSc; Gayer-Anderson, Charlotte, PhD and Quigley, Harriet, MD et al.

C. Mays, Jeffery and Newman, Andy. 'Nation's First Supervized Drug Injection Sites Open in New York'. *The New York Times*, November 30, 2021.

Impact of an Unsanctioned Safe Consumption Site on Criminal Activity, 2010-19. *Drug and Alcohol Dependence.* Vol. 220. March 1, 2021 (last accessed June 15, 2022).

Acknowledgements

I am grateful to my patients and their families for providing me with fresh insights and for sharing with me their conflicts, travails, despondency and delight. I am thankful to Dr Atul Ambekar and Dr Bhaskar Mukherjee for their professional inputs.

Thanks are due to Preeti Gill for taking this book to publishers and to Vineetha Mokkil at Speaking Tiger Books for her astute editing.